Penguin Handbooks
The New Penguin Slimnastics

GW00493357

Diana Lamplugh was born in 1936 and is married with four children. With Pamela Nottidge, Diana developed Slimnastics, specializing in a positive approach to health through exercise, sensible eating, preventive medicine and tension control. From study and experience over a number of years of different groups of women (and some men) of all ages, she has researched the effect of Slimnastics on the relief of overstress. Diana teaches many Slimnastics groups in adult colleges and she also teaches swimming for both children and adults.

Pamela Nottidge was born in 1931 and is also married with four children. She obtained a diploma in Physical Education, Theory and Practice, at Bedford College of Physical Education and has taught in South Africa, Canada and Great Britain. Pamela initiated Slimnastics in England. She has designed the most successful Slimnastics exercises, specializing in exercises not only for fitness and slimming but also for the relief of tension. She teaches physical education to physiotherapy students at a London teaching hospital.

Slimnastics is a method of fitness and relaxation and the Slimnastics movement was founded by the authors in 1964, starting with small groups at home. Diana Lamplugh and Pamela Nottidge have written two previous books, *Slimnastics* (Penguin) and *Stress and Overstress*. The advice in this book is primarily intended for individuals, but group support is helpful and there are hundreds of enthusiastic groups in many parts of the country. The Slimnastics movement is non-commercial, promoted by the Slimnastics Association, a non-profitmaking organization. More information can be obtained from: The Slimnastics Association, 14 East Sheen Avenue, London SW14.

The New Penguin

SLIMNASTICS

A Guide to Good Living

Diana Lamplugh and Pamela Nottidge

Penguin Books

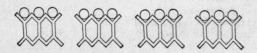

Penguin Books Ltd, Harmondsworth,
Middlesex, England
Penguin Books, 625 Madison Avenue,
New York, New York 10022, U.S.A.
Penguin Books Australia Ltd, Ringwood,
Victoria, Australia
Penguin Books Canada Ltd, 2801 John Street,
Markham, Ontario, Canada L3R 1B4
Penguin Books (N.Z.) Ltd, 182–190 Wairau Road,
Auckland 10, New Zealand

First published by Penguin Books 1980
Copyright © Diana Lamplugh and Pamela Nottidge, 1980
All rights reserved

Typeset, printed and bound in Great Britain by
Hazell Watson & Viney Ltd,
Aylesbury, Bucks
Set in Monotype Times Roman

To the members of our Slimnastics groups and the many professional people in the medical world who have been so enthusiastic about Slimnastics.

Contents

List of Figures   11
Acknowledgements   14
Diana Lamplugh Introduces You to Slimnastics   15

PART I   EXERCISE FOR FITNESS   19

Chapter 1   Exercise and the Body   21
Muscles and Movement   21
The Joints of the Body   28
Understanding Your Back   31

Chapter 2   Exercises for Fitness   37

Posture   37
Head, Neck and Face   40
Shoulders and Arms   43
Hands and Wrists   47
The Chest   50
Spine and Trunk   54
Pelvis and Hips   57
The Knee   60
Feet and Ankles   63

PART II   FOOD FOR FITNESS   69

Chapter 3   Food for Health   71

Individual Needs   71
How Many Calories Do You Need?   73
Striking a Balance   74
Eating to Suit Yourself   80
Some Different Approaches to the Weight Problem   81
How About You?   84
The Food-for-fitness Eating Guide   92
The Food-for-fitness Calorie Tables   94

Chapter 4   Cooking and Eating for Fitness   103

The Golden Rules for Healthy Cooking   104
'Sensual' Cooking   108
Herbs and Spices   109
Cook to Suit Your Pocket   114
Nourishing Meals Throughout the Day   116
Salads   127
Recipes   128

PART III   RELAXATION FOR FITNESS   143

Chapter 5   What is Stress?   145

How to Recognize Overstress   146
The Nervous System   148
'Fight or Flight'   151
Problems Caused by Tension   152

Chapter 6   Introducing the Slimnastics Relaxation Programme   154

The Neuromuscular Relaxation Programme   155
Positive Ways to Blow Off Steam   157
Sleep – the Most Complete Form of Rest   168
Quietening the Restless Mind   170

PART IV   FITNESS IN SICKNESS AND IN HEALTH   173

Chapter 7   Take Care of Yourself Day by Day   175

Skin   175
Body Odour   177
Halitosis (Bad Breath)   178
Hair   179
Teeth   180
Eyes   181
Ears   181
Hands and Nails   182
Take Care of Yourself on Holiday   182
Take Care of Yourself in Extremes   183

Chapter 8   Take Care of Yourself and Others Throughout Life   185

The Menstrual Cycle   185
Pregnancy   193
Post-natal   195
Babies   199
Toddlers   199
Children   202
Teenagers   206
The Menopause   207
Maturity   212

Chapter 9   Take Care of Yourself in Sickness   220

What is a Heart Attack?   220
Early Detection of Cancer   224
Recurrent Ailments   225

Chapter 10   Taking Care of Others in Emergency   234

Be Prepared – The Emergency First-aid Cupboard in the Home   234
Help – Emergency!   235

PART V SLIMNASTICS FOR YOU   243

Chapter 11   The Slimnastics Ten-week Fitness Plan   245

Introducing the Ten-week Fitness Plan   246

Chapter 12   Course of Exercises for Groups   248

The Slimnastics Class   248

Appendixes

1. The Fitness Circuit Chart   293
2. Approximate Number of Calories Per Day Needed at Different
   Life Stages   294
3. Approximate Number of Calories Per Minute Needed for
   Various Activities   295
4. Personal Statistics Chart   296
5. Ideal-weight Charts (for Women and Men)   297
6. Conversion Table for Weight   298
7. Your Personal Diet Sheet   300

List of Figures

1. Human Skeleton, Front View — 22
2. Human Skeleton, Back View — 23
3. Muscles of Human Body, Superficial Layer, Front View — 24
4. Muscles of Human Body, Superficial Layer, Back View — 25
5. Correct Body Posture — 39
6. Exercises for the Head, Neck and Face — 41
7. Correct Posture of the Head and Neck — 42
8. Exercises for the Shoulders and Arms — 45
9. Exercises for the Hands and Wrists — 48
10. Exercises for the Chest — 52
11. Exercises for the Spine and Trunk — 55
12. Exercises for the Pelvis and Hips — 59
13. Exercises for the Knee Joint — 61
14. Exercises for the Feet and Ankles — 65
15. High Kicks for Low Spirits — 161
16. Desk Exercises — 162
17. Sequence at the Kitchen Sink — 163
18. Car Exercises — 164
19. Strap-hanging on the Tube Train — 165
20. Exercises in Bed — 166
21. Loo Exercises — 167
22. Premenstrual Tension — 189
23. Exercises with Partner — 192
24. Post-natal Exercises — 197
25. Mother and Baby — 200
26. Mother and Child — 203
27. Tummy and Spare Tyre (Abdomen) — 211
28. Post-hysterectomy Static Exercises for Abdominal and Pelvic-floor Muscles — 213
29. Exercises in the Bath — 216
30. Easy Exercises for Stiff Joints — 218
31. Shoulder-joint Exercises — 219
32. Emergency First Aid — 240
33. Daily Stretching Exercises — 252

12   List of Figures

34. Stretching Sequence   253
35. FITNESS COURSE OF EXERCISES   Fitness 1   254
36. Fitness 1 (cont.)   255
37. Fitness 2   256
38. Fitness 2 (cont.)   257
39. Fitness 3   258
40. Fitness 3 (cont.)   259
41. Fitness 4   260
42. Fitness 4 (cont.)   261
43. Fitness 5   262
44. Fitness 5 (cont.)   263
45. Fitness 6   264
46. Fitness 6 (cont.)   265
47. Fitness 7   266
48. Fitness 7 (cont.)   267
49. Fitness 8   268
50. Fitness 8 (cont.)   269
51. FITNESS CIRCUIT   Fitness Circuit – Part A   270
52. Fitness Circuit – Part B   271
53. Fitness Circuit – Part C   272
54. Fitness Circuit – Part D   273
55. EXERCISES FOR THE BODY   Head and Neck Exercises   274
56. Ribcage and Back Exercises   275
57. Chest and Breast Exercises   276
58. Shoulder-girdle Exercises   277
59. Spine and Hip Exercises   278
60. Shoulder and Thigh Exercises   279
61. Knee-joint and Thigh-muscle Exercises   280
62. Hip and Pelvic-girdle Exercises   281
63. Abdominal Muscle Exercises   282
64. Trunk-muscle Exercises   283
65. Hip-joint Exercises   284
66. Upper Spine and Shoulder Exercises   285
67. Spine and Hip Exercises   286
68. Hip Exercises   287
69. More Hip Exercises   288
70. Abdominal Muscle Exercises   289
71. Hip Mobility Exercises   290
72. Hip and Buttock Exercises   291
73. Free-standing Exercises   292

Acknowledgements

We are very grateful to all those who have acted as consultants, advisers and contributors and would like to thank them for the time, energy, expertise and thought they have given in the preparation of this book.

Part I, Chapters 1 and 2: Dr Robert A. Billings, M.B., M.R.C.P., M.R.C.G.P., hospital practitioner, rheumatology; Dr M. Rennes, lecturer at University College Hospital Medical School; Violet Palmer, former Vice-Principal, St Mary's Hospital School of Physical Medicine (she is a physiotherapist and a physiotherapy teacher).

Part II, Chapter 3: Elizabeth Morse, Senior Scientific Officer to the British Nutrition Foundation; Jane Davies, Community Dietician for Wandsworth; Diana Jotcham, Dietician to the Ealing Group of Hospitals.

Chapter 4: Adrienne Sackin, gourmet cook and the Lunch-time Group; Jane Davies, Community Dietician for Wandsworth; Anne Battle, teacher of home economics.

Part III, Chapters 5 and 6: J. Macdonald Wallace, Principal Lecturer in Health Education, West London Institute of Higher Education; Dr Desmond Kelly, psychiatrist at Atkinson Morley Hospital (an authority on anxiety and depression); Dr Hannah Jones, community medicine, Porthcawl.

Part IV: Dr Michael Smith, Hon. Chief Medical Officer to the F.P.A. and a consultant in preventive medicine; Dr George Brown, G.P., The Health Education Council; Dr Karin Jardine Brown, G.P. and lecturer in first aid; Margaret Davies, beautician.

We would also like to thank our Slimnastics leaders and the members of their classes who contribute so much enthusiasm and ideas, and in particular, the members of the Slimnastics groups under the Ealing Further Education Authority and Richmond Adult College for testing all the ideas in this book.

Diana Lamplugh Introduces You to Slimnastics

Slimnastics combines exercise, tension control and healthy eating. It is a practical and positive approach to fitness and relaxation of both body and mind. The group, within which Slimnastics is most often taught, encourages the achievements of each individual, promotes discussion and exchange of ideas, and assists the group members to help themselves and support each other.

Since 1964, and particularly since the publication of our first book *Slimnastics* and the follow-up *Stress and Overstress*, the Slimnastics movement has grown enormously. We have found that our concept of total fitness provides the answer for which so many people, both young and old, have been searching. We now have many professional Slimnastics leaders who take groups for the adult and further education authorities and other organizations. The demand for these classes has been constantly increasing and their existence is encouraged by the health authorities and community dieticians. There are, too, countless home groups practising Slimnastics and many brave people who have the perseverance and tenacity to stick to a fitness programme on their own.

However, it is not only the Slimnastics movement which has grown; our own knowledge of our subjects has deepened and widened. As we searched, researched and learned, we became more and more aware of how much there was to add since we wrote the previous books. For example, Pamela has been teaching physical education to physiotherapy students at a London teaching hospital, and I have been working in two adult education colleges. Many of my students experience joint and muscle problems. I talked these over with Pamela and she in turn discussed them with the physiotherapists. Together we sorted out and sifted the ideas they put forward so that I could pass on to my students those which were relevant, easy to put into practice and safe to try without supervision. We began to realize that specialized medical knowledge could be of inestimable help if it were generally available, not only in aiding the afflicted but also in preventing problems in the first place.

In 1975 I attended an extra-mural course on neuromuscular relaxation, given by the University of London. This form of tension control suited Slimnastics as though tailor-made – it is completely unhampered by mumbo-jumbo, easy to teach and rewarding to learn. I began to notice the difference in myself as well as my students as soon as I introduced tension control (as we call it) into my Slimnastics classes. They too began to report back to me easier home lives, improved attitudes to work and better health. I received accolades from doctors for reduced blood pressure, cholesterol levels, etc. This combination of exercise, sound nutrition and tension control made Slimnastics a complete approach to total fitness. We passed on our ideas to our leaders and they had equal success.

Pamela also taught anatomy at 'The Place' which is the London home of the Martha Graham School of Dancing; I studied psychology, group therapy and first aid. All these courses were invaluable, but we decided when writing this book not to rely only on our own knowledge and experience but also to consult and take advice from experts in every field; not one expert but two or three, as occasionally their ideas would conflict or be too clinical. It was our job to bring the ideas together and to make sure they both worked in practice and were acceptable as well. This is where our classes and those of our leaders were such a great help.

However, we knew that it was not only important to write a book containing information which would be applicable to a wide cross-section of people and become an essential part of their daily lives, but also to ensure that everyone would want to read it, understand the facts and advice and, most important of all, put them into practice.

We started with the bones, the joints and the muscles as these are parts of the body we can instantly do something about – even if it is only for the moment! We can do a few exercises, we can look in the mirror and check our posture. It is fairly simple to react and feel the benefits of exercises. We also know how widespread, debilitating and depressing pain can be, which is why we have taken each part of the body in turn and given explanations of pain and have shown how to help oneself both instantly and in the long term. Just reading these sections should encourage everyone to do the exercises which may help to prevent trouble in the first place.

By the time you have read Part I, Exercise for Fitness, you will realize that good posture is most important. If the body is out of balance, something will go wrong. Excess weight is one of the chief causes of that imbalance and it also puts an extra strain on the internal workings of the body. We think that the realization that excess weight and poor diet increase stress should encourage the reader to approach Part II, Food for Fitness, with an open mind.

In our experience most people find it almost impossible to be objective about the food they feed themselves – they have been conditioned from an early age and tend to believe what they want to believe and only hear what they want to hear! Nutrition is a much more complex subject than magazines would lead us to believe, so we have tried to spell it out as clearly as possible. We have divided it into two chapters – how to eat for good health and then the 'good news', how to enjoy it! Our ideas for 'sensual' cooking, which appeal to the senses of taste, sight, smell and feeling, are for everyone who loves good food.

Much of the harm we do ourselves through straining our bodies or over-eating is the result of uncontrolled tension, leading to 'over-stress'. Our method of relaxation and tension control is straight-forward, using the effect on the brain of releasing the tension in the muscles. Once learned it can be put into operation at any time and in any place and will help you not only to reduce the pressures you are putting on yourself but also to make the most of the mental and physical abilities you already have. Often we are unaware that we are under tension, so we hope that by the time the readers have been through the first two parts, they will understand that Part III, Relaxation for Fitness, also applies to them.

Part IV, Fitness in Sickness and in Health, deals with skin, hair, teeth, body odour, the body-changes (which can be baffling, dis-concerting and frustrating not only to people experiencing them but also to people around them), first aid and general health (all those niggling ailments which can be such a trial but often do not seem to merit medical attention). We could not leave these out in a book which aims to help you to become completely fit.

Naturally we cannot avoid some diseases but we hope to encourage you to have the strength to withstand any onslaught. A 78-year-old member of one of our groups who had to have an operation to remove a polyp from his rectum, was pronounced by the hospital doctor to be in an 'excellent state of fitness'. His weight, good nutrition, suppleness and calm frame of mind will stand him in good stead during the months ahead.

The last part of the book shows you how to put all these thoughts into *action*. We give you an easy to follow ten-week programme which will only take a few minutes a day plus about an hour each week. You can do this on your own or get together with a group – weighing, measuring, exercising, controlling tension, reorganizing your diet and cooking with pleasure – all this adds up to balanced living. You have only to meet members from our Slimnastics groups to know that it works.

Each chapter of the book has been sent to two or three separate experts in that particular field. They have contributed to these chapters, commented on and approved every word that has been written. Pamela has again produced some excellent exercises which are easy to follow and really work.

All these ideas and exercises have been tested fully and during the past nine months in particular. I see about 200 people every week in my twelve Slimnastics groups held by the Ealing Further Education Authority, Richmond Adult College and at my home. The age range is from 15 to 82 but of course we include some pregnant mothers, babies and toddlers. There are too few men but the numbers are increasing. The members of my groups are so patient, tolerant and have so much sense of humour that I often feel that it is I who gain most from the classes. To all of them I am very grateful.

Part I
Exercise for Fitness

Our sedentary, civilized lives no longer fulfil our biological
need for exercise. We have to take positive steps to remedy
the situation. Even those of us who already lead active
lives need exercises to improve our physical health and
appearance and to relieve nervous tension.

This does not mean, however, that you have to rush
straight out and run round the park or go for a work out in
the nearest gymnasium. Neglected muscles need to be
re-educated gradually to strength and tone; joints must be
eased back to full mobility with regular exercise. The
exercises in this part are designed to improve slowly but
steadily muscle strength and endurance, flexibility and
mobilization of the joints and spine and to help circulation
and co-ordination. These exercises will also promote deeper
breathing and relaxation.

Exercise tenses and relaxes two types of muscles. The first
group are the voluntary muscles, which are used for
movement and over which we have full control. Muscles
which are automatically exercised at the same time are the
involuntary groups such as the digestive tract, skin and
blood vessels. This means, for instance, that every chest
exercise helps to get rid of superfluous fat, improving the
overall shape of the body, and also increases the capacity
of the lungs and strengthens the heart. Exercises which
bring elasticity back to slack and sagging tummy muscles at
the same time hold the internal organs in position. These
groups of muscles will, as a result, perform better, easing
such chronic conditions as constipation or indigestion.

After completing a few exercises one invariably feels
refreshed and relaxed, with renewed vigour and a clear alert
mind. The reason for this is not solely because of improved

circulation and increased oxygen intake but is also because we have taken active steps to relax our muscles. When one group of muscles contracts, those which are in opposition have to release their tension. You can see this clearly when you bend your elbow so that your hand can touch your shoulder. While the inner group of muscles is contracting hard to pull your hand inwards, the group on the outside of your arm has to relax or your hand would be unable to move.

All voluntary muscles have the dual power of contraction and relaxation. However, living muscle never becomes completely relaxed, but is constantly in a condition of slight contraction, the degree of which varies with the state of health of the individual. This is known as muscle tone or tonus. Fully-exercised muscles gain tone and are able to hold the posture of the body more naturally and easily. It is very exhausting, as well as unsightly if your head is thrust forward, your shoulders stoop, your back is rounded and your tummy protrudes. A well-balanced body can work without strain.

With exercise, sleep patterns also improve. Although everyone suffers from the occasional difficult night, a person with a well-exercised body is far less likely to suffer from regular bouts of insomnia. A relaxed sleep helps to recharge the batteries.

It's never too late to start doing exercises. The elderly who include exercises in their daily routines become not only fitter but seem younger in every way. The exercises increase the strength and mobility of their limbs and joints, their circulation and co-ordination improves and the stimulation of their glands, particularly the adrenal, helps them regain some of their youth and confidence.

In Part I we look at the body as a whole, and the joints, muscles and back in particular. We analyse not only their functions in isolation but also in relationship with each other and the part exercise has to play in improving mobility, strength, endurance and shape. We hope to prove that exercise improves the quality of life as well as prolonging it.

Chapter 1
Exercise and the Body

The *skeleton* (see Figs. 1 and 2) is the framework to which the muscles are attached. The muscles clothe the skeleton, give it shape, maintain its posture and cause it to move. The joints are the means by which movement takes place.

The harmonious working of muscles and joints influences the internal working of the body. The circulation of the blood (everyone has approximately eleven pints or six litres) is affected by activity. The rate of the heart-beat and of breathing is affected by exercise; as is the working of the digestive system and of all other internal organs of the body.

The *muscles* on the outside of the body (see Figs. 3 and 4) can be made to work at will. These voluntary muscles account for a third of the weight of an adult man. The muscles inside the body, such as the heart, the digestive system, the uterus, work involuntarily. Therefore we can control our bodies by using the outside muscles in order to place the limbs and trunk in a position suitable to the occasion, and keeping them there for as long as is necessary. This is only possible if the muscles are kept in good condition by being used regularly and correctly to maintain their strength. This cannot be achieved unless the *joints* are in good condition, so it is essential that they are moved daily as far as they will go, and are not allowed to become stiff.

Muscles and Movement

There are three main effects of regular muscular exercise – increased *skill*, *strength* and *endurance*. These effects are to a large extent the results of different processes and they are to some degree capable of being independently developed.

The increase in *skill* and co-ordination which comes with repetition

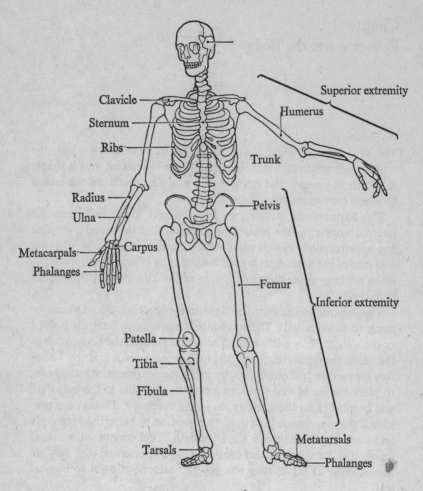

Clavicle

Sternum

Ribs

Radius

Ulna

Metacarpals

Phalanges

Superior extremity

Humerus

Trunk

Pelvis

Carpus

Femur

Inferior extremity

Patella

Tibia

Fibula

Metatarsals

Tarsals

Phalanges

Fig. 1
Human Skeleton, Front View

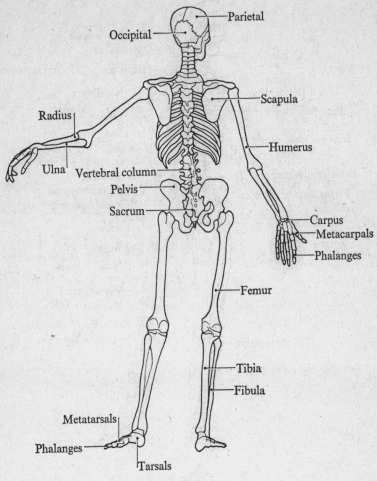

Parietal

Occipital

Scapula

Radius

Humerus

Ulna

Vertebral column

Pelvis

Sacrum

Carpus

Metacarpals

Phalanges

Femur

Tibia

Fibula

Metatarsals

Phalanges

Tarsals

Fig. 2

Human Skeleton, Back View

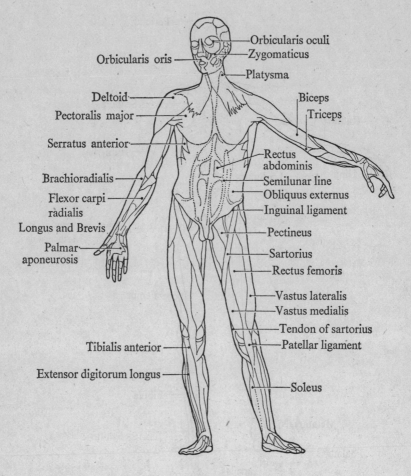

Orbicularis oculi
Zygomaticus
Orbicularis oris
Platysma

Deltoid
Pectoralis major
Biceps
Triceps

Serratus anterior

Rectus abdominis
Brachioradialis
Semilunar line
Flexor carpi radialis
Obliquus externus
Longus and Brevis
Inguinal ligament
Palmar aponeurosis
Pectineus
Sartorius
Rectus femoris
Vastus lateralis
Vastus medialis
Tendon of sartorius
Tibialis anterior
Patellar ligament
Extensor digitorum longus
Soleus

Fig. 3

Muscles of Human Body, Superficial Layer, Front View

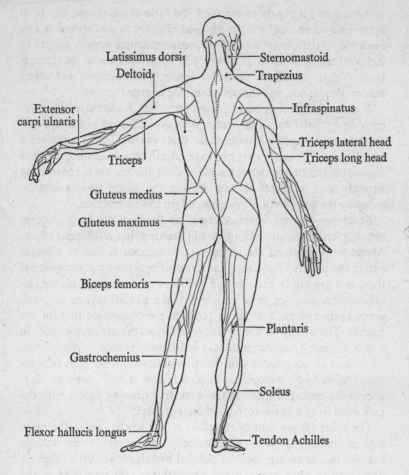

Latissimus dorsi
Deltoid
Sternomastoid
Trapezius

Extensor
carpi ulnaris
Infraspinatus

Triceps lateral head
Triceps long head
Triceps

Gluteus medius

Gluteus maximus

Biceps femoris

Plantaris

Gastrochemius

Soleus

Flexor hallucis longus

Tendon Achilles

Fig. 4

Muscles of Human Body, Superficial Layer, Back View

of movements is poorly understood and little physical basis has been uncovered to account for the obvious changes in performance. The evidence to date suggests that the neuromuscular system adapts to repeated movements by removing the control of those movements from higher conscious levels to lower, subconscious and more automatic systems, and this speeds up the muscle responses.

Muscle strength can be increased by either graded strength exercises or by brief maximal work. A major effect of either type of exercise is to increase muscle bulk. Brief maximal work requires a speedy release of energy, which occurs during the anaerobic phase of muscle contraction which takes place while the muscle is contracting strongly and is therefore compressing the blood vessels and so reducing the amount of oxygen needed for the contraction.

Endurance-training exercise, such as medium to long distance running, cross-country skiing, or hill walking, has a different effect. About 50 per cent of the increase in endurance is due to changes within the muscle. The size of the muscle fibres does not increase but there is a growth in the size and numbers of mitochondria, the cellular components of muscles which make use of oxygen to break down carbohydrate and fat to produce the immediate fuel for the muscle. The ability to use fat is increased to the greatest extent. In addition there is an increase of a red-muscle protein – myoglobin, which has an oxygen-carrying function in muscle which can be compared to that of haemoglobin in blood. This is easily seen by comparing the dark red meat of the wild, free running rabbit with the pale meat from a hutch-reared sedentary rabbit.

The other 50 per cent of the effect is due to changes in the heart and circulatory system. Paradoxically, while short-term intense exercise causes enlargement of skeletal muscle, it has little effect on heart muscle other than to allow it to withstand transiently increased blood pressure. However, endurance-training exercises cause an enlargement of the heart, allowing a greater volume of blood to be pumped at each beat, and thus involving a greater blood-flow through muscles during exercise. In addition, the dilatation of capillary vessels in muscle (including heart muscle) increases – again allowing greater delivery of blood to working muscles. These adaptations to exercise may also have a beneficial protective effect against cardiovascular disease – certainly endurance-trained athletes run a low risk of heart disease.

The beneficial effects of exercise in promoting growth of muscle tissue is often overlooked by designers of slimming regimens. Dietary calorie restriction alone causes a loss of body fat but also causes a loss of muscle protein, the effects of which contribute to the feeling of lassitude and weakness often reported by slimmers.

Regular exercise stops this loss of muscle protein and the accompanying loss of strength, tone and endurance of muscle. And remember, any foodstuffs which are diverted to form new muscle protein are thereby unavailable for conversion into fatty tissue, so that fat deposits should waste proportionately. Incidentally, there is also evidence that regular exercise actually *decreases appetite*, especially if performed just before mealtimes.

Muscular injuries caused by inappropriate exercise

In persons unaccustomed to exercise, forced muscular work often results in muscle pain during exercise, and a lasting tenderness or stiffness of the muscle. Very little is known of detailed cellular causes of these symptoms, but they are associated with accumulation of acid waste products in muscle, loss of potassium from muscle and swelling due to accumulation of fluids from the bloodstream. Usually the symptoms clear up with rest and continuing moderate exercise, but acute muscle soreness which can cause lameness requires complete rest, since it probably results from a breakdown of protein within the muscle. In addition to problems associated with muscle itself, unaccustomed vigorous exercise can cause stretching and tearing of tendons and ligaments, particularly those of antagonistic muscles, and especially during work where the muscles are being stretched as they contract, such as running downhill or lowering heavy weights.

The prevention of all of these conditions is simple. Avoid sudden intense exercise without first 'warming up' and keep clothing on until the muscles are warm. Cold muscles, with a low blood-flow, have no option but to break down local energy stores without the use of oxygen, and large quantities of acid waste products accumulate quickly. Allowing the muscle sufficient time to increase its blood-flow to a high level before increasing the workload literally warms up the muscle so that it works faster and supplies blood-borne fuels and oxygen in amounts adequate for sustained work. Conversely allow time to wind down at a low workload after intense exercise – don't just stop dead. This avoids a strain on the heart and also allows the blood flowing through muscles to flush away waste products more efficiently.

Of course it is also common sense not to attempt too big a task. There is no point in running to the point of exhaustion just to be crippled by muscle soreness for the next week. Make all progress in duration and intensity of exercise gradual and this need never happen.

The Joints of the Body

Without joints our bodies would be incapable of movement. There are several types of joints in the skeletal system and they are highly sophisticated and durable. With the exception of the large weight-bearing joints of the hips and knees they give relatively little cause for trouble.

The joints of the limbs and the trunk are called *synovial* joints which allow free movement in a wide range. There are three types:

(a) Ball and Socket Joints. These allow movement in all directions over a wide range. These are the hip and shoulder.

(b) Hinge Joints. The two major hinge joints of the body are to be found in the knees and the elbows. Movement of these is limited. The elbow joint cannot be bent backwards and the knee joint cannot be bent forwards.

(c) Gliding Joints. Typical examples of these are to be found in the intervertebral joints of the spine and in the foot. These allow a limited range of movement.

Damage to the joints

'Wear and tear' injuries to the smooth cartilage lining the joints occurs in most people, leading in some cases to arthritis (osteo-arthrosis). These changes, normally associated with ageing, may be produced prematurely in young people who overuse, or severely injure their joints, and can produce ballet dancer's ankles or hurdler's knee.

Joints depend for their function on the stability provided by their surrounding ligaments and muscles, and injury to these 'soft tissue' structures can be just as important in causing early joint damage. Continued 'trauma' to a joint may result in either the breakdown of the smooth cartilage to a roughened joint surface, or the formation of scar tissue within the joint ligaments, the result of which is loss of elasticity and full range of movement. When a joint loses its full mobility as a result of an injury, any movement will be painful, and excessive force will lead to a breakdown of the scar tissue with the resulting recurrence of the old injury, thus establishing a vicious circle of increasingly disabling injuries.

Treatment for damaged joints

Any injury around a joint must be treated in the first instance by the reduction of swelling and by immobilization. This can be done by elevating the injured part, applying a cold compress (ice cubes in a plastic bag, wrapped in a towel) for short periods, and then strapping the joint with a firm (but not too tight) bandage. Any severely injured joint should be X-rayed for fracture.

While the joint is painful it should be rested; in the case of the ankle and knee, crutches can often be helpful to avoid putting weight on the joint. Since the joint needs to return to a full range of painless movement, exercises supervised by your doctor or physiotherapist must be started early and very gently to ensure that permanent stiffness does not set in. Home treatment with hot water immersion and regular stretching exercises is frequently sufficient to achieve a good result quite quickly. Full activity must not be resumed until the joint is functionally as good as the same joint in the opposite limb.

Many common ailments such as a frozen shoulder, tennis elbow and sore heels are not in fact due to problems within the joint, but to injured muscle and tendon attachments, and often disappear with rest. If the symptoms persist, you should consult a doctor.

Arthritis and rheumatism

These require serious attention. They are terms used to cover many different conditions, all of which cause pain and disability. Ten per cent of the world's population is afflicted by arthritis and two million people in the U.K. experience some form of rheumatic complaint each year. Children can develop one of the various forms of juvenile arthritis, whereas in adult life the onset of arthritis is most likely to herald either osteoarthrosis or rheumatoid arthritis.

Osteoarthrosis

Osteoarthrosis is a 'wearing out' of the joint, with destruction of the smooth cartilage, narrowing of the joint space, eventually leading to destruction of the underlying bone. In most cases it occurs simply as a slightly stiff and painful joint which needs little in the way of treatment, whereas more extreme cases may require physiotherapy. Severely damaged joints such as the hip or knee can be replaced with artificial joints, providing a new lease of life free from incapacitating pain and stiffness.

Rheumatoid arthritis

This disease develops in the lining membranes of the joints as an inflammation causing pain and swelling, followed by erosion of the cartilage and bone. Afflicting some half-million adults in the U.K. and possibly as many as ten thousand children, it is an unpredictable disease which in its mildest form may cause only vague aches and pains, and in its most severe can progress to a rapid destruction of joints with gross disability, even death.

Early diagnosis and treatment of this disease have been improved considerably in recent years. Aspirin is no longer the only 'corner stone' of therapy, instead a new generation of anti-inflammatory drugs has arrived, and for those with a more active form of the disease, then treatment with, for instance, Gold can provide many with a dramatic remission of symptoms. As with osteoarthrosis, surgery is used today to repair and replace damaged joints, allowing the arthritis sufferer to continue leading an active life.

The do's and don'ts of arthritis

1. Do protect the painful swollen joint from overuse – you can only make things worse by trying to 'work off' the pain.
2. Don't allow the joint to remain immobilized over long periods. Rest and splinting are helpful, but all joints should be put through their natural range of movement three or four times daily.

3. Do ask your doctor to supply adequate doses of analgesics, or anti-inflammatory drugs to kill the pain, as this will enable you to keep your mind on other activities.
4. Don't submit to arthritis, it can easily lead to depression and acceptance of disability. Instead, get your doctor to make a diagnosis and outline a plan for treatment and rehabilitation. Prescribed exercises will play an important part and should be carefully thought out and performed regularly.
5. Do remember to go 'out and about' and participate in as many recreations as is possible. This is important to avoid developing the 'crippled mentality' that can be more destructive than the disease itself.
6. Do shed any excess weight and don't allow yourself to put it on again as this will lead to more problems with your joints. Find a satisfying diet suited to your daily activity and calorie requirements (see Part II, Food for Fitness).

If you have any particular joint problems you will find more detailed information in the following sections together with ways to alleviate the 'wear and tear' and take more 'care'.

Understanding Your Back *Dr Robert Billings*

The back is a complex piece of organic engineering, enabling man to stand erect and undertake a wide variety of movements including lifting, bending and turning. The foundation stones of the back are the twenty-four vertebrae, seven of which are in the neck (cervical), twelve behind the chest (thoracic) and five in the low back (lumbar). They are suspended between, and cushioned by, tough intervertebral discs and they are also stabilized on either side by small sliding (facet) joints which link one vertebra to another, permitting a small degree of movement of the one upon the other. Movement of the whole spine such as turning to look over one's shoulder, will involve a small movement at each level. Any block to the movement of a small joint by injury or arthritis will be felt as pain at that level in the back and there will be difficulty in completing the movement.

Each vertebra has a boney arch posteriorly, acting as a protective tunnel for the delicate spinal cord and its nerve roots, two of which emerge at each level, on either side of the spine close to the disc.

These small nerves wind around the body providing the sense of touch, and the sensations of pain and vibration. They also enable impulses from the brain to control muscles at that level. A nerve may become trapped by a damaged disc or bone and symptoms of pain, numbness or weakness will be felt in the appropriate region of the body. The commonest 'nerve root syndromes' are those of fibrositis in the shoulder, pain in the arm and pain down the back of the leg known as sciatica. Occasionally the symptoms of a trapped nerve may simulate chronic migraine, middle-ear trouble, heart pain (angina) or gastro-intestinal problems, and even a ruptured appendix. There are many patients who have had investigations and even major operations for these symptoms only to find later that the problem arose from the spine.

The intervertebral disc consists of a central gelatinous pulp surrounded by a tough fibrous ring, which is bound tightly to the vertebrae above and below. Each disc acts as a shock absorber, and without them the spine would be a rigid structure unable to absorb the impact of the great loads created by straining, sneezing, lifting, etc. The disc of a child has a largely fluid centre with a closely knit outside ring. As the disc ages the contents start to solidify into a 'crab meat' consistency, the outer ring losing its closely knit cohesion, and finally in the fourth and fifth decades the pulp becomes hardened and indistinguishable from its outer ring. With this ageing process the disc slowly loses its ability to provide a cushioning effect for the spine, and itself becomes liable to injury.

The disc is designed to withstand certain loads, but certain spinal postures and activities can alter the pressure considerably within a disc. The least pressure occurs when one lies in bed, and increases when standing upright, reaching its maximum on standing with legs straight and bending the upper part of the body forward to lift a weight. Such pressure may become too great for a disc and the central pulp bursts out with great force, either up into the body of the vertebra above, or out through the ring into the spinal canal. It is here that it may press on a nerve root, causing sudden severe pain – this is the true 'slipped disc'.

The stability of each vertebra depends upon the integrity of the posterior arch to which are attached the powerful back muscles. Recent studies have demonstrated that this arch may be broken either by a sudden severe injury such as a sharp twist of the spine or by constant repetitive strain on the vertebra, which may occur in athletes or gymnasts. This leads to a 'stress fracture'. A break in the arch allows the vertebra to become unstable and the disc to become weakened by movement, which in time leads to a situation of recurrent back pain. These fractures are often missed by the standard X-ray techniques, and only an oblique view of the spine will demonstrate this painful defect.

There are also the soft tissue injuries which occur when muscles or ligaments in the back are bruised or ruptured. These are no less painful and may cause as great a disability as an injury to bone, disc or joint.

Acute back pain

These problems of soft tissue injury, slipped disc, blocked facet joints and boney arch fractures are probably responsible for the majority of 'mechanical' failures in the back. They frequently have a sudden onset following an injury or after lifting a weight badly. There can be few people who have not experienced the agonizing pain in the back with muscle spasm associated with one of these lesions. The best immediate treatment is to rest the back in a comfortable but well supported position, take tablets for the relief of pain and apply warmth to the painful region with a hot water bottle.

The majority of these acute problems resolve themselves in a matter of hours or days, and as soon as the pain and the muscle spasm has subsided light activities can once again be resumed. It is worth thinking about the original cause of the pain – it might be postural, or follow an exhausting training session or an awkward lifting action. Whatever the cause analyse the movements which led to the injury and use the experience as a lesson to prevent further recurrences.

Persistent back pain

Should the acutely painful back fail to settle down, or should other symptoms develop in the arms or legs, then it is time for further investigation of the problem. Your doctor will have made his own assessment and may advise further rest on a hard mattress with the addition of stronger pain relief tablets and muscle relaxants. If any other treatment such as manipulation, traction or spinal injection of corticosteroid drugs is to be done, then X-rays of the spine and occasionally blood tests will be done at this stage.

Manipulation of the spine is now carried out not only by osteopaths and chiropractors but also by some general practitioners and hospital specialists. The results of manipulation depend upon the correct manipulation being applied at the correct level of the spine at the correct time.

Traction is sometimes helpful in relieving back pain associated with pain down the leg. This acts by distracting the vertebrae, thus drawing in the bulging disc. Corticosteroid injections with local anaesthetic frequently give great relief of pain by reducing the inflammation, swelling and muscle spasm at the site of injury.

Persistent back pain should always be investigated to exclude the other diseases which may affect the spine.

Ankylosing Spondylitis is predominantly a disease of young men. It involves increasing pain and stiffness in the spine, which is particularly severe in the mornings. This may be diagnosed by X-ray changes in the sacro-iliac joints with calcification of the spinal ligament. Recently, a sophisticated blood test known as the HL–AB27 Antigen has been developed to diagnose this condition and has shown that this form of back pain is genetically inherited. The importance of making an early diagnosis in this condition is that the treatment in the painful phase is the reverse of that recommended for mechanical back problems. If sufferers are treated with bed rest, traction, corsets etc. then their spine becomes irreversibly stiff and painful. Early diagnosis with a programme of spinal exercises can help their spine become supple and free of pain.

Every doctor should be aware that back pain may have a more sinister cause, and unless early investigations are done it is possible to miss spinal infections and tumours and these can progress rapidly unless treated. X-rays remain the traditional method of visualizing the spine, but more modern techniques of bone scanning can provide evidence of bone disease such as an enlarging secondary deposit from a cancer of the breast, long before the changes become evident on plain X-rays.

Emotional problems are frequently blamed as the cause of back pain, yet while people with backache have been found to be more anxious than non-sufferers there is little evidence that they are more depressed than others. Much of their anxiety stems from their inability to 'throw off' the back pain and return to a normal active life.

Pregnancy and the back

During pregnancy, hormones act on the joints and spine to make them more supple and lax. While this is an advantage for the growth and birth of the baby, it does cause back pain in almost half the women. Not only does the extra weight of the baby cause a postural strain, but the stretching of the abdominal muscles leads to weakening of spinal support both in pregnancy and afterwards. The combination of lax spinal joints with weak abdominal muscles predisposes the young mother to mechanical injury from simple tasks such as lifting the baby from the cot.

Those most 'at risk'

The 'at risk' groups of people include therefore the nursing mother, the overweight, those with a previous history of back pain, the physically unfit, and those people whose occupation or recreation creates excessive strains on the spinal column such as dockers and weight-lifters.

Prevention of back pain

For all these people, and indeed for all those who have not yet suffered from back pain, there are a few guidelines which will help in the prevention of back pain:

LIFTING

1. Never stoop to pick up a weight, always keep the back straight, the knees bent and keep the weight as close as possible to the body.
2. If something looks as though it might be too heavy, don't 'have a go' instead call for assistance.
3. Heavy weight-lifting has been shown to be a hazardous pastime

for the amateur leading to some of the most severe back problems
– it is better to avoid it as a training activity.

POSTURE

1. A comfortable erect posture is not only graceful but will also help prevent early 'wear and tear' in the spinal discs and joints.
2. The spine is under least strain when supported in its natural lines of curvature. This means that back supports in cars and chairs should mould comfortably to the spinal outline.
3. Whatever one's job it should not be necessary to stoop with a curved back over the work. This leads to postural back pain. Situations of this sort can be remedied by raising the working level and regularly moving about instead of standing or sitting in a fixed position.
4. A firm mattress is essential, since it maintains the spinal contours during sleep.

PHYSICAL FITNESS

1. Avoid obesity – this adds unnecessary loading to the spine leading to early arthritic changes.
2. Keep the abdominal muscles strong by regular exercise. Tightening of these muscles occurs when one strains downwards and a similar exercise can be done in any situation such as at work, or driving, etc. These muscles are essential in controlling spinal stability.
3. Regular exercise which does not cause the back to ache is to be encouraged. Discontinue any activity which regularly causes pain. This is particularly applicable to children undergoing severe training routines for sport. Back pain in children or adolescents must never be ignored and the provoking cause must be removed. Injury to the growing spine, like the growing sapling, can lead to permanent deformity when fully grown.

Chapter 2
Exercises for Fitness

Posture

Good posture is your best self-advertisement. You will not only look poised and confident, you will probably feel it too. If you are standing, sitting, moving and lying correctly there will be less strain or stress on the muscles, ligaments or joints and this will prevent fatigue and pain. Good carriage is also essential in order to allow all your vital organs plenty of room in which to function; breathing also becomes easier and deeper.

With bad posture you probably not only look tired and defeated but feel that way too! After all, the weight of your limbs, head and trunk will be dragging on the muscles, causing continual strain on the joint structures and ligaments. If you are balanced you will not feel the weight of the head, limbs or trunk. In the following pages you will notice again and again how often poor posture can be the root cause of our aches and pains. Unfortunately most of us neglect our posture until some trouble forces us to stop and take stock. However, we hope that you will realize that a small amount of effort now could save you much distress in the future.

What is good posture?

Look at the diagrams of the skeleton on pages 22–3 (Figs. 1 and 2), and see the way the head is balanced on the neck, the curves of the spine, the pelvic girdle, the legs, knees and feet. Hang a tape measure down the centre of a full-length mirror. Standing sideways, the plumb-line should fall from the top of your head, through the ear-lobe, shoulder, middle of the waist, centre of the hip joint, behind the kneecap and in front of the ankle bone.

Face the mirror and look at yourself.

Are your eyes level or is your head on one side, thrust forward or pulled back?

Are your shoulders level, hunched forward or pulled back?

Are your tummy muscles pulled in, ribcage lifted, and buttocks firm? (Are you still breathing?!)

Are your knees together? (See the Knee, p. 60.)

Is your weight balanced over the ankles? Are they together?

Developing good posture

Good posture begins in bed. Your mattress should be firm. If necessary, place a board underneath it to prevent sagging. Use a small pillow for your head. When resting lie flat on your back; occasionally turning on to your stomach, with your feet over the end of the mattress, hips and knees straight, stretch your arms above your head (elbows bent if necessary).

Excess weight puts extra strain on the muscles and joints. Weight control is essential for good posture.

Exercise is also important. To hold a good position easily and naturally the muscles need to be strong and all the joints flexible.

Whatever you are doing (see Fig. 5), you must balance all parts of your body evenly to eliminate strain. Gradually good posture will become a habit.

The following routine will balance your body correctly:

1. Pull up the arch muscles of the foot so that the weight is carried evenly on the heel and the outer border, the forefoot gripping the floor, the knees slightly bent.

2. Tilt the pelvis so that the stomach muscles are held up and contracted with the buttocks tucked under and the buttock muscles firmly contracted. (Stand with a 'rock-bottom and pinch-proof posterior instead of a sag-back with prominent belly' is how one textbook puts it!)

3. The shoulders should be slightly up, the chin tucked in, and the head balanced on the shoulders so that there is no tendency for the head to fall forward.

Practise this regularly and you will achieve one of the best aids to health, both of body and mind.

Correct Body Posture

Good Posture	Fig. 5	Bad Posture
	Standing	
	Sitting	
	Lying	
	Lifting	
	Putting on shoes	
	Ironing	

Head, Neck and Face

A balanced position of the head and neck is important if one is to maintain good posture. Try to become constantly aware of how you are holding your head and neck. If you thrust your head forward, this may indicate that you need your eyes testing. If you hold your head on one side when you are talking to people or listening check that your hearing is not at fault. When you have eliminated any basic causes for poor posture make every effort to stand, sit, move and lie so that the head is perfectly balanced above the spine. Constantly check yourself – look in mirrors, shop windows, any reflection (it's not for vanity, it's for your health!) – gradually it will become natural. Remember that eventually you will discover that it is much less of an effort to stand up straight than slumping with the muscles under tension and strain.

Exercises for the head, neck and face (see Fig. 6) are needed to mobilize the joints and strengthen the muscles. Because most movements we make with our bodies involve the head and neck, it is essential that we keep these joints supple or the whole trunk will be tense and stiff. The first set of mobility exercises will loosen all the small joints of the vertebrae in the neck and gently use the muscles of the neck.

The second set of exercises are those to strengthen the muscles of the neck so that they can hold the head on the shoulders without fatigue and strain. This will improve your posture and help balance and control the rest of your body. Strengthening and easing the tensions of the facial muscles gives the face more youth and shape, firming the sagging jaw line and smoothing away the wrinkles. Those of you who are losing weight will need to exercise away that double chin! and firm the neck line.

Activities which exercise your head and neck

At home: cleaning windows, stretching to high shelves, decorating and painting (remembering to move the head constantly and not cause tension by holding the neck in one position for any length of time).
At play: ball games.

Exercises for Head, Neck and Face

Fig. 6

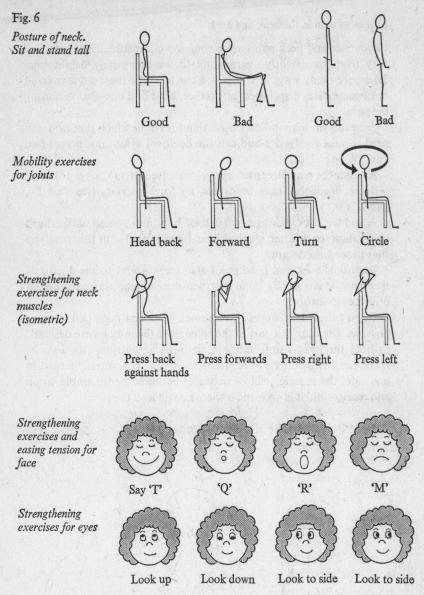

Posture of neck. Sit and stand tall

Good   Bad   Good   Bad

Mobility exercises for joints

Head back   Forward   Turn   Circle

Strengthening exercises for neck muscles (isometric)

Press back against hands   Press forwards   Press right   Press left

Strengthening exercises and easing tension for face

Say 'T'   'Q'   'R'   'M'

Strengthening exercises for eyes

Look up   Look down   Look to side   Look to side

Causes of pain in the head and neck

Headaches and neck pains are a common complaint. The effects can vary from the slightly aggravating to the completely debilitating. There are many ways in which you can alleviate these pains yourself or in some cases dispel them altogether. First find out what is causing the pain.

A headache may indicate illness and fever in which case you will need to take analgesics and call the doctor if symptoms persist (see Part IV, page 230).

A headache may be caused by eye strain (see Part IV, page 181).

Some headaches may be caused by food allergies (see Part IV, page 226).

A sudden neck pain may be caused by injury – such as the head being flung back after a car accident (whiplash) – in this case you should see your doctor.

Persistent neck and head pains also merit a visit to the doctor as they can be caused by bone destruction, vascular abnormalities or other complications.

One of the basic causes of recurrent head and neck pain is poor posture. The neck is a part of the spine; and the muscles are designed to hold the head comfortably in the upright position (see Fig. 7). If the head is thrust forward, leans back or is consistently tipped to one side, the muscles will of necessity be under considerable strain and tension and it is no wonder that this will lead to pain.

Correct Posture of the Head and Neck

Fig. 7

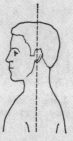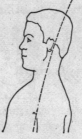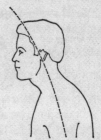

Good – correct upright position

Bad – hollow back, head back

Bad – round shoulders, head thrust forward

The other common cause of pain in this part of the body is physical tension caused by mental stress. Tense hands on the steering wheel in a traffic jam can result in a stiff and aching neck or headache. Frowning or lifting the eyebrows can cause a tense scalp. If tension is the reason for your pain you should take the advice in Part IV, Relaxation for Fitness, as well as in this part.

Immediate self-help for relief of pain

You need warmth and rest. Have a long warm bath. Lie on your back with a folded warm towel under your neck. Stay there for 20 minutes to half an hour listening to the radio or practising your neuromuscular relaxation (see Part III, page 155). A soluble aspirin can be taken if desired.

If you are unable to have a bath and short bed rest, fold the warm towel lengthways until it looks like a scarf. Wind this firmly round your neck and secure it with a safety pin. This will support the head and allow the muscles to rest. You can also make a collar out of a stocking filled with foam rubber, or, if you need a really firm support, a rolled up newspaper. These aids will ensure that you are carrying your head in the correct position without strain.

Shoulders and Arms

We use and abuse our shoulders and arms constantly. We lift heavy weights, lift carelessly, push prams and trolleys, drive cars, stoop over desks, tense over typewriters and machinery. Our joints and muscles need to be very flexible and strong to withstand this tension and strain. Correct use of these limbs is very important to prevent back trouble.

Caring for your shoulders and arms

Study your posture. Rigid shoulders cause muscular tension, uneven shoulders put a strain on the back, and round shoulders contract the chest and lead to limited breathing with the consequent strain on the lungs and heart.

Make sure your working conditions are free from muscular strain. During the Second World War a survey into factory machinery and its effect on the body produced concrete evidence that repetitive tasks, implements at the wrong level and any work requiring constant physical tension not only produced muscle strain with consequent illness and loss of manpower but also discontent and bad work. Unfortunately this report was shelved at the end of the War, and even now only enlightened firms, principally in Scandinavia, Japan and the U.S.A., consider this aspect of work important.

Look at the diagrams concerned with posture (see Fig. 5 on page 39). These will show you ideal sitting and working positions. It is advisable to take frequent and regular short breaks to do one or more of the mobilizing exercises (see Fig. 8). You will then be able to work longer and harder without harming yourself. The mobility exercises will keep your joints supple; the strengthening exercises (see Fig. 8) will help hold the shoulder girdle strongly on to the outside wall of the ribcage. When your muscles work efficiently your general posture will improve. Choose two exercises in each section and do them for a few minutes each day.

Activities which exercise your shoulders and arms

At home: polishing, cleaning windows, scrubbing floors, hanging up the washing, painting and decorating, reaching top shelves.
At play: ball games such as tennis, netball, volleyball or quoits.

Causes of pain in the shoulder and arms

Pain in the joints can be caused by injury or inflammation and should be checked by a doctor.

A 'frozen' joint (one which is not achieving full movement) also needs medical attention – see The Joints of the Body, page 29.

Bad posture (round shoulders, uneven shoulders and those which are rigidly drawn back) is the most frequent cause of a pain in the lower neck and shoulders. Round shoulders can result from poor posture due to rigid hip muscles which tilt the pelvis forward and force the person to curve the small of his back and hunch his shoulders in order to maintain balance while sitting or standing. Round shoulders can also be the outward sign of asthma sufferers or they

Exercises for the Shoulders and Arms

Fig. 8

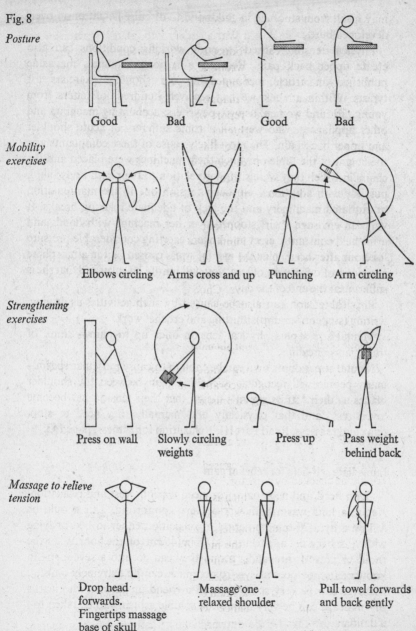

Posture

Good   Bad   Good   Bad

Mobility exercises

Elbows circling   Arms cross and up   Punching   Arm circling

Strengthening exercises

Press on wall   Slowly circling weights   Press up   Pass weight behind back

Massage to relieve tension

Drop head forwards. Fingertips massage base of skull   Massage one relaxed shoulder   Pull towel forwards and back gently

may result from stooping in childhood to disguise height or an over-developed bust.

Physical tension caused by poor working conditions can also create upper back pain. Recently a national women's magazine published an article recommending our shoulder exercises for typists. Within a week we had received hundreds of letters from young girls and women, using typewriters, accounting machines and other appliances, who were all chronic sufferers of acute shoulder and upper back pain. The most likely cause of these complaints was the height of the table on which their machines were placed and the chairs in which they were sitting in relation to their own body build, possibly with additional muscular tension due to the manipulation of outdated machinery and the lack of adequate relaxing breaks. If you can envisage a girl stooped over her machine with hands and arms held constantly erect and fingers exerting considerable pressure for hour after hour, plus the mental stress caused by the atmosphere and noise of open-plan offices, you will hardly be surprised that she is suffering at the end of the day.

Physical tension can also be caused by such activities as driving, writing (students' cramp), knitting and crochet work.

Mental stress plus physical tension adds up to pain – think of traffic jams or exams.

Mental stress on its own can be enough to cause muscular spasm – many people will recognize an aching pain between the shoulder blades as their 'stress signal'; a sign that their tension has become 'overstress' and that physically and mentally they need to stop, relax and reassess. Read Part III, Relaxation for Fitness, page 143.

Immediate self-help for relief of pain

As with head and neck pain, you need warmth, rest and relaxation. Again, a long warm bath will be very comforting. This should be followed by a 20-minute period of relaxation either in bed or lying with your back flat and feet raised 18 in (46 cm) off the floor. When the shoulder muscles are under strain they can go into a severe spasm known as scapulocostal syndrome and it can be extremely painful. Massage can be very soothing, and a friend or partner who learns this massage can be very helpful. A soluble aspirin can be taken too if desired.

Hands and Wrists

No man-made machine has yet been made which can compete with the range of movement and expression of which our hands are capable. Unfortunately it is just because so many joints and muscles are involved that this area of our body can cause pain and suffering.

Caring for your hands and wrists

Help your hands by doing the exercises (see Fig. 9). If you study them carefully you will realize that many of your daily chores can become mobility exercises for the joints or strengthening exercises for the muscles. Choose the ones which suit you best.

Activities which exercise your hands and wrists

At home: screwing, unscrewing, opening doors, wringing out clothes or dishcloths, sewing, tieing shoelaces, doing up buttons, typing, peeling vegetables.
At play: pottery, weaving, knitting, handicrafts, playing the piano or other musical instruments, golf, tennis.

Causes of pain in the hands and wrists

Read the doctor's article, The Joints of the Body, on page 28.

See your doctor about any swelling of the hands or joints and he will investigate the cause and advise on treatment. Also consult your doctor if your wrists or fingers are painful and stiff (particularly in the morning) and if you are losing your grip. It is important to establish the cause as treatment can be very different.

Take seriously any injury, however slight, to your hands or wrists. Neglect can set up trouble for the future.

As our hands are at our extremities, it is here that poor circulation will be most apparent particularly in cold weather. This can be painful and unsightly.

'The hands are the mirror of the soul,' they say! Unless you are very practised at concealing your emotions, it is more often than not with your hands that you will display your tensions. Skin rashes, finger fidgets and nail biting all say something about you!

Exercises for the Hands and Wrists

Fig. 9

Posture. Resting wrists and hands

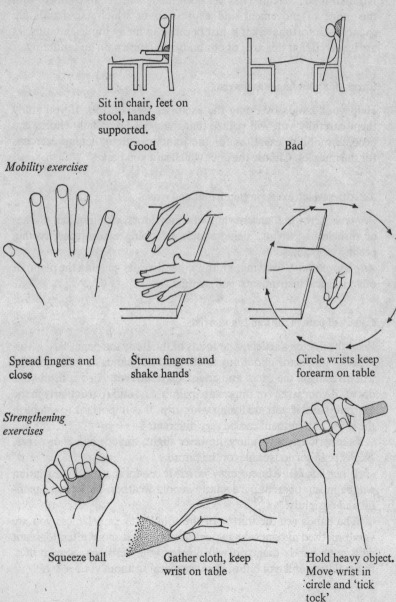

Sit in chair, feet on
stool, hands
supported.

Good   Bad

Mobility exercises

Spread fingers and
close

Strum fingers and
shake hands

Circle wrists keep
forearm on table

*Strengthening
exercises*

Squeeze ball

Gather cloth, keep
wrist on table

Hold heavy object.
Move wrist in
circle and 'tick
tock'

The skin of the hands is often a sensitive guide to allergies.

The nails can give clues to the diagnosis of ten or more serious medical complaints (e.g. anaemia, arthritis, heart and liver disease).

Immediate self-help for relief of pain

Heat helps to relax tense muscles and is often soothing to inflamed joints. Bathe your hands for five minutes in warm water and then massage each hand with cream; this will improve your skin, and circulation and gently exercise the joints and muscles.

Very inflamed joints which are red, painful, swollen and stiff, particularly in the mornings, need complete rest. If the inflammation is allowed to subside there is every chance that no harm will be done to the joints and they will return to normal. The hand with inflamed joints (particularly in rheumatoid arthritis) should be rested flat, not curved. Physiotherapists frequently make splints which immobilize and support the inflamed and painful joints, while still enabling the hand to function. The hand and inflamed joints should be put gently and passively through a full range of movements several times daily to prevent stiffness and disability.

If you have injured your hand in any way – for instance jarred your thumb, fallen on your wrist, caught a ball awkwardly – the best instant treatment is immobilization and an ice pack. This can be made by filling a plastic bag with ice cubes from the refrigerator; tie securely and remake as necessary. This will reduce the bruising and swelling which will further damage the joint. Keep the pack really cold with fresh ice until you have had professional help. Carry out this procedure even with a young child – a damaged joint at any age can cause problems in the future.

If you suffer from poor circulation, exercise not only the hands but the whole body. Never forget to wear warm, wind-proof gloves when you go out in cold weather. When you return to a warm atmosphere, keep moving. Immerse your hands in warm water or preferably have a warm bath followed by a warm drink. Whatever you do, never sit huddled over a blazing fire with hands outstretched or lean with your hands behind you on a hot radiator. Both seem tempting but your hands will become even more painful and may develop chilblains and cracked skin.

If nail biting is your problem, there are commercial preparations

N.P.S. – 4

which will help you by making the taste quite foul. Read Part III on relaxation and tension relief. If you want to make constructive use of finger fidgets buy one of those adult games made especially for people like you. They look beautiful and are excellent exercise for your hands. Alternatively you might take up the piano, guitar or harp.

Hand disabilities

For those with disability in their hands or wrists, unable to undertake various personal, household or gardening tasks, there is a wide range of aids available. In the U.K. these are on display at the Disabled Living Foundation, 346, Kensington High Street, London W14 8NS.

The Chest

The skeleton of the thorax forms a protective cage round those vital organs – the lungs and the heart. This is no rigid structure but a beautifully constructed piece of engineering with flexible cartilages and articulated joints which allow the muscles to move the ribs and expand the thoracic cage, so that as we breathe in and our lungs fill with air, the volume is increased. As we expel the air the intercostal muscles relax, allowing the ribcage to retract. Normally we repeat this process about 15 to 20 times per minute. Your respiration rate depends on your age, sex and activity, but it is faster in children and women, and for everyone it is increased with activity.

We breathe for two reasons. First, we need to inhale air to supply oxygen to the blood which circulates and feeds the cells, organs, glands and nerves; the brain also needs a constant and plentiful supply of fresh oxygen without which we simply cannot think clearly. Secondly, we need to exhale air to rid the blood of waste products. Deep breathing improves our metabolism which breaks down the food and creates energy. Exercise can greatly improve the vital capacity of the lungs and give an increased mobility to the chest walls.

It is essential to strengthen and tone up the muscle of the heart with gradual but consistent exercise. The heart is an extremely efficient muscle acting as a central pump which keeps about 11 pints (6·3 l) of blood in constant circulation around our body. By beating on average 72 times a minute, one drop of blood does a complete circuit in one minute. As with other muscles of the body, systematic exercise will strengthen the heart. This means that a slower heart-beat is a sign of fitness, giving the body more blood and yet using fewer heart-beats. Again, as with other muscles of the body, if the heart is under-exercised and in poor condition, sudden pressure may cause strain and even bring on a heart attack. (This is discussed more fully in Part IV, page 220).

Caring for your chest

The diseases associated with the heart and chest, namely coronary thrombosis, lung cancer and chronic bronchitis, are some of the major causes of death in the western world. Nowadays this fact applies almost as much to women as to men.

Smoking is a major cause of thrombosis and bronchitis. One in ten of all heavy cigarette smokers will ultimately develop a lung cancer. If you smoke and care at all about its effect on your chest – you must use all your willpower to give it up. If you find that quite impossible, at least change to a low-tar brand and do not inhale.

We need constantly to practise the mobility exercises (see Fig. 10) in order to encourage and maintain the flexibility of the joints of the ribs and the vertebrae of the spine. Choose two of the exercises and do them regularly. Deep breathing too is an exercise. Many of us simply do not know how to breathe. We do not exhale properly and leave much of the stale air and impurities behind.

Try this exercise: half fill a glass with water and with a straw exhale the air from your lungs until the water stops bubbling. Inhale with short breaths of air and repeat. Do this three times each day (not more or you may feel dizzy). You will soon teach yourself to breathe more deeply, freely and easily. It is the exhalation which is important. You will automatically breathe in deeply if all the stale air has been removed.

The strengthening exercises (see Fig. 10) are essential too not only for the heart but also to maintain a good posture which will enable the thorax to work efficiently. Choose two of the strengthening exercises to do daily.

The incidental but satisfying by-product of these exercises is the way they improve the external muscles of the chest! Although they

Exercises for the Chest

Fig. 10

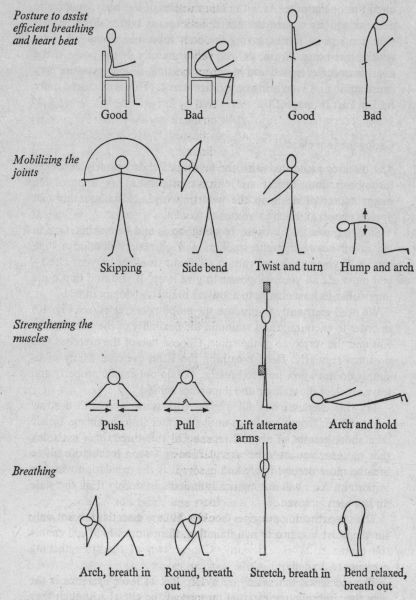

Posture to assist efficient breathing and heart beat

Good   Bad   Good   Bad

Mobilizing the joints

Skipping   Side bend   Twist and turn   Hump and arch

Strengthening the muscles

Push   Pull   Lift alternate arms   Arch and hold

Breathing

Arch, breath in   Round, breath out   Stretch, breath in   Bend relaxed, breath out

will expand the measurements of the male chest, they will not increase the size of the bust – but they will improve your shape!

It is quite obvious from our Slimnastics groups that the size of their busts can cause more stress to women than practically any other part of their anatomy. From the very start of puberty a young girl can suffer quite severely either from being over-developed or flat-chested.

The bust consists of glands covered by fatty tissue; it is a passively mobile, superficial structure lying on the pectoral muscles. Pregnancy, excess weight and hormones or plastic surgery will increase the size of the bust; it may be decreased by slimming or an operation. Nothing can be done to improve the size or shape of the breasts themselves through exercise alone. However it is possible to strengthen and tone the muscles surrounding and supporting the bustline. This will give you an uplift and improve your outline! If you want to be assured that the exercises are actually working, do them naked in front of the mirror and watch the effect!

Activities which exercise your chest

At home: walking upstairs, gardening. Anything which makes you breathless.
At play: swimming, jogging, running, team games (any sport which makes you out of breath). Exercises using weights.

Pain in the chest

The sudden onset of pain in the chest always merits medical attention. It may turn out to be muscular spasm caused by mental tension but it is much better to be safe than sorry.

Check your posture. Muscular tension in the chest can be traced to the poor posture of the shoulders and neck. For instance if your posture is uneven, with one shoulder higher than the other or one shoulder more forward than the other, the effect may be reflected in the chest.

Anxiety, stress and excitement can cause spasm in the chest and shortness of breath. Read Part III, Relaxation for Fitness, and practise releasing tension from the muscles as well as deep breathing.

Immediate self-help for relief of pain

Calm down. A short time spent in controlled, slow and deep breathing can do much to dispel anxiety. If possible, stand by an open window, shoulders relaxed, breathing through your nose to warm the air, and filter dust and germs. Concentrating on the ribcage, expand it sideways, forwards and upwards, depressing the diaphragm and pushing out the abdomen. Breathe as deeply as possible without raising your shoulders and then exhale through both nose and mouth. Pant for a few seconds at the end of the exhalation to remove as much stale air from the lungs as possible. Breathe in and out a few times in this manner and you will then feel calm and collected.

Even if the pain or chest condition is of organic origin it is essential to remain as quiet and unfussed as possible while waiting for medical help. Panic or stress can only aggravate the situation. Your fears may well be unfounded, so take it easy!

Spine and Trunk

If you are unfit, overweight and suffering from tension, your back is most likely to be at risk. Almost more working hours are lost per year from back trouble than for any other reason. This is hardly new: there is evidence of bad backs in Egyptian mummies 5,000 years old, and even in prehistoric monsters. Unfortunately many of the reasons for backache and pain are not fully understood and consequently much research is being done and advice and treatment vary alarmingly. However, you can reduce the risk of back pain or help to alleviate it once it has occurred.

In the first place it is essential really to understand your back and this is very well described in the article on page 31. You will begin to realize the utmost importance of maintaining the mobility of the spine by positive toning and relaxing exercises. The movement between two adjacent vertebrae is very limited but it is considerable in the spine as a whole. Any pain in the back will cause the whole body to appear stiff and awkward (see Fig. 11). You need to flex, extend and rotate in order to strengthen the muscles of the back and keep the many joints flexible.

Exercises for the Spine and Trunk

Fig. 11

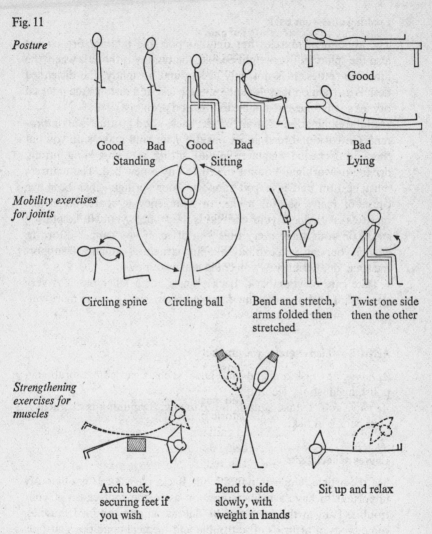

Posture

Good Bad   Good Bad

Standing   Sitting

Good

Bad

Lying

Mobility exercises for joints

Circling spine   Circling ball   Bend and stretch, arms folded then stretched   Twist one side then the other

Strengthening exercises for muscles

Arch back, securing feet if you wish   Bend to side slowly, with weight in hands   Sit up and relax

Looking after your back

The abdominal muscles not only support the internal organs but also the spine. In overweight people, the tummy is the area where the fat often settles. It is not only ageing and unsightly, the distended flesh is a strain on muscles and on the back, and distorts the internal organs so that they are unable to function properly.

In the elimination of strain on the back, good posture is all important. Go back and read about posture again and make sure you put this into operation whenever you are sitting, standing, lying, lifting, driving or working. You may need to buy a new bed. The mattress must be firm and give you support. Poor springing has been the cause of many painful backs. In emergency a board under the mattress is a help. If your car seat is the trouble you will be putting strain on your spine every time you drive. If you cannot afford to change your car, you can buy webbing structures which will support the back, or alternatively you could make your own.

Take care of your back. Back pain is not a killer but it is very unpleasant and once having damaged your back you are more vulnerable another time.

Activities which exercise your back

At home: any task on hands and knees such as gardening, scrubbing, polishing, dusting, decorating.
At play: golf, tennis, squash and dancing. Swimming is excellent if your back is at risk.

Causes of back pain

See the article, Understanding Your Back, page 31. It is obviously important to have a medical opinion as to the root cause of your trouble. Pain in the back can be due to fatigue, strained muscles, some types of arthritis, disc trouble and medical conditions such as kidney and gynaecological disorders.

Immediate self-help for relief of pain

If the pain is very severe ask the doctor to come to you. While you are waiting, keep warm and lie flat. If your mattress is soft ask someone to put a board underneath it to make it more firm. One doctor insists all his back patients lie for 20 minutes in the hour flat on the floor in a sleeping bag. He has excellent results.

Try to work out the immediate cause of the onset of pain. It is important to try to pinpoint the movement or position which triggered off the attack, so that you can avoid it in future. Once you have 'done in your back' the same cause is more than likely to have the same effect another time.

A survey undertaken by physiotherapists at a well-known teaching hospital established that many of their back patients had good strong healthy muscles and joints but their injury had occurred doing a movement which they had done many times before, but on this occasion at a time of particular physical or mental stress or after a bout of flu. We can underestimate the amount of strength an infection can sap from the healthy body, and antibiotics can lull us into ignoring the necessary period of convalescence.

When you have seen your doctor, take his advice and put it into operation. Only if this does not work should you seek another opinion. As there are so many opposing views, trying two cures at once may well cancel each other out! Some people swear by osteopaths and chiropractors, others try acupuncture, a psychological approach or a change of diet, different drugs, plaster supports or physiotherapy. All these cures have worked for some people in varying degrees.

When your back is getting better the question often asked is whether or not one should exercise. If your back is still hurting, a rule of thumb is to stretch gently. If this relieves the pain, you can start very slowly doing other exercises which do not hurt. If stretching increases the pain, rest the back and do not start exercising until the pain has disappeared.

Pelvis and Hips

The pelvic girdle is a very strong structure which transmits the whole weight of the body to the legs. The two hip bones are fused to each other and to the backbone and this surrounds the bladder, rectum and reproductive organs. All these organs have openings through the pelvic-floor muscles, consequently these muscles have to be very strong to hold these organs all in position. The pelvis itself is immoveable except in women during childbirth and all movements must take place from the lumbar spine or at the hip joint.

It is into the deep hollow on either side of the pelvis that the head of the femur fits to form the ball and socket joint of the hip.

Looking after your pelvis and hips

Many people are very concerned about the shape of their hips, buttocks and thighs. Unfortunately, we can do nothing to improve our bone structure and although excess weight is not inherited, we do inherit the tendency for the fat to settle in certain areas and particularly on the hips and thighs. We need to make every effort to lose that excess weight but it is also essential to do exercises to firm up flabby muscles and give them some shape.

The gluteal muscles, together with fat, form the roundness of the buttocks. They contract to extend the hip joint when you are running and climbing upstairs and they raise the body from stooping or sitting. They also maintain the balance when walking and running by keeping the pelvis level as weight is transferred from one leg to the other. It is important to keep the muscles of the hips and buttocks and the muscles down to the knee fit and strong as they are in constant use. If they are weak and under-exercised they will cause fatigue and exhaustion. Regular exercising of these muscles will help not only looks but general health.

The mobility exercises (see Fig. 12) will keep your hip joints and lumbar spine loose and flexible. The strengthening exercises for the muscles will not only improve the shape and tone, they will also break down any deposits of fat and relieve any tension. Choose two from each section to do every day.

Activities which exercise your pelvis and hips

At home: climbing stairs, gardening. Any tasks which require bending and lifting (from knees and hips with straight back).
At play: walking, running, jogging (especially uphill), cycling, swimming, rowing, riding, skiing, golf, skipping, athletics, putting the weight.

Exercises for the Pelvis and Hips

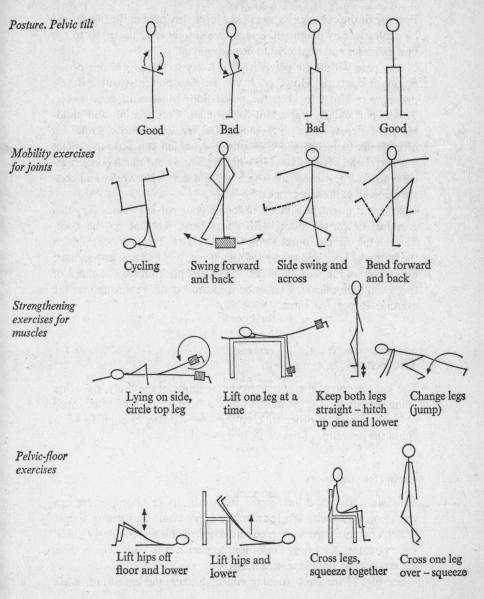

Fig. 12 With each exercise, harden buttocks, press knees together, and pull up pelvic-floor muscles between legs.

Posture. Pelvic tilt

Good Bad Bad Good

Mobility exercises for joints

Cycling Swing forward and back Side swing and across Bend forward and back

Strengthening exercises for muscles

Lying on side, circle top leg Lift one leg at a time Keep both legs straight – hitch up one and lower Change legs (jump)

Pelvic-floor exercises

Lift hips off floor and lower Lift hips and lower Cross legs, squeeze together Cross one leg over – squeeze

Pain in the pelvis and hips

Because of the complex nature of the joint, any pain in the hip should be professionally diagnosed and advice sought (and taken) as to the best exercises and treatment to be undertaken.

Any pain within the pelvis itself is likely to arise from one of the organs it contains. However, it will help to prevent trouble if you make every effort to keep the pelvic-floor muscles in good order. This is particularly important for women. Constipation and childbirth put a great strain on these muscles. Weakness or overstretching often leads to incontinence or prolapse, which can seriously affect our social and sexual lives. No woman should need much encouragement to do a few exercises which will aid sex, waterworks and constipation all at the same time!

At first it might be difficult to locate your pelvic muscles. Try this exercise: lie on the floor, with knees bent, feet flat on the floor. Tighten the tummy muscles and press the back into the floor; tighten the buttocks hard and then press the knees, legs and ankles together; now draw up the muscles inside. Hold this position for the count of three and then release. Remember to keep breathing throughout the exercise. Repeat five times.

The Knee

The knee is one of the two major hinge joints of the body, the other being the elbow. It is the muscles of the thigh which need to be toned up by exercises in order to keep the knees strong enough to withstand the pressures of the whole body weight.

Caring for your knees

You can understand how much strain obesity or poor posture can put upon this joint. We must make every effort to get our weight under control if we wish to avoid knee problems. Similarly check your posture; the knees are often the part of the body which show the strain of an unbalanced carriage.

See Fig. 13 for strengthening and mobilizing the knee joint. Walk

Exercises for the Knee Joint

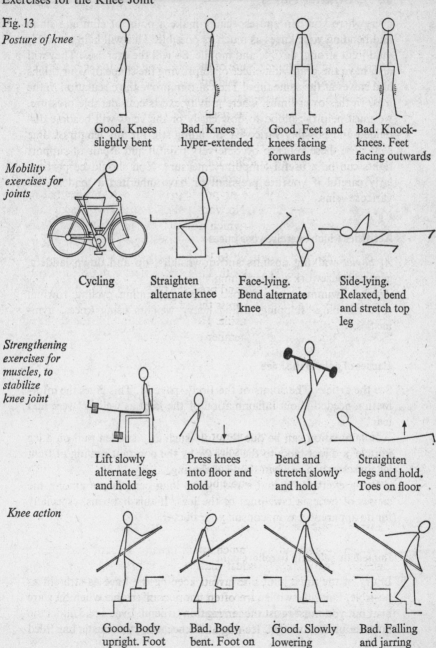

Fig. 13
Posture of knee

Good. Knees slightly bent

Bad. Knees hyper-extended

Good. Feet and knees facing forwards

Bad. Knock-knees. Feet facing outwards

Mobility exercises for joints

Cycling

Straighten alternate knee

Face-lying. Bend alternate knee

Side-lying. Relaxed, bend and stretch top leg

Strengthening exercises for muscles, to stabilize knee joint

Lift slowly alternate legs and hold

Press knees into floor and hold

Bend and stretch slowly and hold

Straighten legs and hold. Toes on floor

Knee action

Good. Body upright. Foot on stair

Bad. Body bent. Foot on edge

Good. Slowly lowering weight

Bad. Falling and jarring

everywhere you can and especially make a point of climbing stairs and bending your knees as much as possible. This will help keep this vital joint strong, flexible and mobile. So will the exercises. They will also have the gratifying effect of improving the shape of your thighs and calves at the same time! They also improve the circulation in the legs. In the lower limbs, where gravity exerts considerable pressure, we must help the blood to flow easily or the veins will become distended and possibly varicosed. Standing still for any length of time can cause these veins to become very painful and a pair of support tights can be a useful temporary measure. You should be particularly careful if you are pregnant or have inherited a tendency to varicose veins.

Activities which exercise your knees

At home: walking upstairs and downstairs, up and down ladders, general housework and gardening.
At play: swimming breaststroke, running, jumping, cycling, rowing, rope climbing, skipping, lifting heavy weights using knees, gymnastics.

Causes of pain in the knee

See the article, The Joints of the Body, page 31. This gives the information needed about inflammation of the joint as well as 'wear and tear'.

Inflammation can be due to injury such as a sudden pull on a leg muscle, a direct blow to the knee or by the constant pulling of tight leg muscles such as when skiing or skating.

Being overweight, and standing for long periods are among the causes of oedema (swelling) of the legs. If this happens, especially for no apparent reason, consult your doctor.

Immediate self-help to relieve pain

Injury of the knee joint needs rest, keeping the knee as straight as possible. Painful, swollen knees are more comfortable when they are bent but you must resist the temptation to bend. Even a pad under the knee should be avoided. Ice-pack the knee using the plastic bag filled with ice cubes, to bring down the swelling so as to avoid any further damage to the joint, and take soluble aspirin for the pain.

Children and young people often injure this joint in sports. They should not be allowed to hobble around regardless but should be forced to rest and apply cold compresses until the swelling and pain have gone, otherwise they will be building trouble for themselves in the future.

Dislocation of the kneecap may require manipulation from the doctor or physiotherapist or it may go back into place spontaneously. In any event it would be wise to check your posture and if necessary seek medical advice as to whether you need special exercises or shoes to correct this dislocation.

Knock-knees and bow legs should be treated in childhood when much can be done to help the child stand correctly.

If you are suffering from osteoarthrosis, avoid obesity, standing or walking for long periods or sitting in one position. Never over-exercise or strain the affected joint. However, it is essential to strengthen the muscles surrounding the joint and you can do this by practising isometric exercises when the knee joint is straight and at rest – push the knee down on to the bed or floor, hold and relax.

Feet and Ankles

The state of our legs and feet is mirrored in our face. If our feet are painful and our legs ache, it will show. Look after your feet for without them we could not stand or walk. However, by using buses, cars and lifts and often doing sedentary work, we neglect these parts of our bodies the most.

Caring for your feet and ankles

Anyone who has suffered from sore and aching feet will realize how vital it is to pay maximum attention to this part of our body. A foot needs strength and stability to support weight and mobility and elasticity for fluid movement and to avoid jarring. Our complex ankle joint needs to be flexible and in good condition to give us ease of movement in running and walking. To achieve this we need to exercise them constantly.

We must not neglect the soles of our feet which are covered with skin and layers of muscles among which lie blood vessels and nerves. The muscles under the arch need strengthening in order to maintain the arch to the correct height (see Fig. 14). Many of the exercises for mobility and strengthening can be practised as you go about your daily lives. Choose two mobility and two strengthening exercises and do them as often as you can.

Bad shoes are the cause of many foot and posture problems. It is worth spending money on footwear. Whatever you do, never slop around in slippers; in fact whenever possible take your shoes off altogether and go barefoot. It is not only good exercise but it gives a feeling of freedom and relaxes the inhibitions!

Pamper your feet. Cut your toe nails and look after the skin of your feet too. Foot sprays or massage with hand cream can eliminate hard ridges on the soles. Adequate foot hygiene and sensible care can prevent athlete's foot which thrives on sweaty unwashed feet! (See Part IV, page 178).

As you get older visit the chiropodist regularly and always go if you are worried about foot problems.

Causes of pain in your feet and ankles

Read the article, The Joints of the Body, page 31.

Injury, sprains, strains, breaks – all deserve immediate medical treatment.

Bunions – when the legs and feet are forced into poor standing and walking positions, various parts of the toes are pressed against the sides and top of the shoe. A bunion can form at the big toe joint.

Plantar Fasciitis – a pain felt in the sole of one or both feet due to inflammation.

Achilles Tendinitis – felt in the heel and calf by ageing sportsmen leading to partial or complete rupture of the Achilles tendon.

Ingrowing toe nails, corns, pressure from hard skin (callosities).

Muscle fatigue caused by flat feet.

Fatigue fractures of the foot.

Sore feet due to weak muscles, athlete's foot, excess weight or oedema (swelling of the ankles and feet).

Bad posture. To turn your feet outwards or inwards upsets the balance and is a strain on the nerves and circulation of the feet.

POOR SHOES!!

Exercises for the Feet and Ankles

Fig. 14

Posture

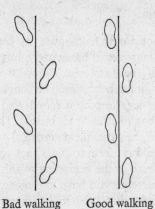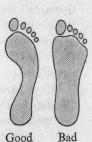

Bad walking   Good walking   One side normal   Good   Bad
Shows weight-bearing part of feet

Mobility exercises for joints

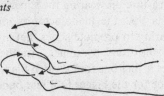

Keep knees braced and legs still. Circle feet both ways

Turn soles inwards and outwards

Bend foot up and down

Strengthening exercises for muscles

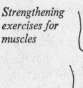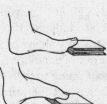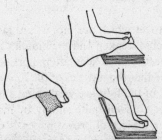

Sitting, keep toes straight. One foot at a time

Grip bean bag with toes curled under

Two heels on floor with feet on book. Lift up to tiptoe

Immediate self-help to relieve pain

All injuries to the ankle and foot should be X-rayed. As you will see from Figs. 1 and 2 there are so many small bones and joints involved that small fractures could easily be dismissed. This will encourage trouble in the future and professional help should be sought as soon as possible. Meanwhile rest the leg, keeping it raised, and ice-pack the swelling (using the plastic bag filled with ice cubes). The doctor will decide the extent of the injury and treatment needed.

Where pain is concerned we always seem to come back to posture. Read again the section on Posture at the beginning of this chapter. Bad posture will destroy any pretence you have to elegance and the appearance of youthful movement; it will also make you more prone to accidents and injury.

Bunions, corns, ingrowing toe nails, bad circulation and sore feet can all be the result of bad shoes. It does not pay to economize or be a slave to fashion where shoes are concerned. Many rebellious teenagers ruin their feet for life by insisting on wearing the shoes of the moment. At last there are signs that the manufacturers are acquiring a conscience and endeavouring to promote shoes that are actually suitable for feet. We hope the trend continues. Another point to remember when buying shoes is that one foot is often bigger than the other. You must buy the shoe for the bigger foot and build the other shoe with a sock. If you have not been doing this you may well have acquired evidence to prove it – your bunion and corns will inevitably be on the bigger foot! Bunions and corns can be temporarily relieved by specially prepared pads which can be obtained from the chemist, but a visit to the chiropodist should not be delayed.

Flat feet which are mobile are rarely painful. The pain occurs as the arches weaken and the muscles become fatigued. If you find that your feet tend to ache after short periods of walking or standing, it may be that the muscles of the foot are out of condition and that the arches of the foot are weakening and beginning to fall. You can test this for yourself quite simply by making a wet footprint after your bath on a piece of brown paper or coloured card. If your print fails to show the customary gap you must practise the foot exercises for strengthening the muscles. Unfortunately if you have had flat feet for some considerable time it is almost impossible to cure them by exercises alone and you should consult your doctor.

Fatigue fractures of the small bones of the foot can occur when there is so much tension on certain bones from muscle pull that the slightest additional force will break the bone. This can happen to young recruits when they go on long marches, to ice skaters and even to joggers – so beware. It is wise gradually to educate your muscles into sustained exercise.

Sore feet or swollen ankles which are due to standing for long periods and to excess weight need rest. Preferably they should be raised. If necessary put a couple of bricks or blocks under the feet at the end of the bed. Make a disciplined effort to lose that excess weight! (Read Part II.)

If your feet and ankles swell up regularly for no apparent reason, consult your doctor.

Part II
Food for Fitness

Chapter 3
Food for Health

Individual Needs

Our health and well-being depend on the food we eat. However, for some people too much food can result in too much weight. Reading through the previous chapter one cannot fail to notice how many times excess weight is mentioned as having an adverse effect on posture, joints, muscles and internal organs. It is impossible to keep our bodies fit and supple if they are hampered by excessive weight. This simple link between nutrition and health is often ignored as can be observed by the extent of obesity among both adults and children.

If you still remain unconvinced that weight does matter, consider the following facts.

The overweight:
are more likely to suffer from high blood pressure and varicose veins,
are more susceptible to diseases of the heart and circulatory system,
may suffer from gall-stones and diseases of the liver and kidneys,
are more prone to develop diabetes and gout,
put extra strain on joints, particularly the hips, knees and spine and osteoarthritis is aggravated,
are more likely to have flat feet and bad posture,
are likely to be more prone to accidents,
if undergoing surgical operations, carry a greater risk and post-operative recovery is hampered,
woman is less likely to become pregnant and excessive weight-gain during pregnancy can lead to complications,
To be 10 per cent heavier than ideal is recognized as a health hazard,
To be 20 per cent overweight is a serious medical handicap.

Add to this the knowledge that excess weight can be ageing, impairing both looks and confidence, and think of the burden we can put upon ourselves! Apart from a few medical causes, the reason for being overweight is too much food!

Slimming down excess weight brings the rewards of regained looks, confidence and vitality; it also improves health. Weight control should be regarded as preventive medicine; when excess weight is lost, health hazards are reduced. If you slim wisely and conscientiously, you will save yourself problems in the future and relieve your doctor of extra work! Slimming does require determination and encouragement but dieting need not be sheer drudgery. We want to prove to you that even when losing weight your food can be interesting and exciting. You will still be able to eat with enjoyment and satisfaction.

Weight is not the only indicator of a good diet. Even those who are not overweight should check the foods they are eating. There is no such thing as a 'perfect' diet and it is in fact easy to survive on a badly chosen, limited food intake. The human being is an adaptable species and can exist on a wide range of foods. There is no one particular food without which we cannot survive, but surviving is not the same as living life to the full.

Increasingly, facts are becoming known about the effect of nutrition on health. Recent medical reports have shown clear links between diet and several diseases of the heart, colon and bowel. The effects of excess food, resulting in obesity, or a deficiency of iron causing anaemia have long been recognized. Many people, though lacking vitality and feeling continuously below par, consider themselves perfectly well because they have forgotten what it is like to feel really fit. Their diet may well be to blame.

As the implications of diet and disease become better understood it is evident that our health and well-being depend not just on *how much* we eat, but on *what* we eat. By putting these theories into practice, eating a varied diet, tailored to our own needs, we can take a positive step towards good health, confidence and vitality.

The food we eat has two essential functions within the body: it provides us with energy and also with the nutrients required to keep the body functioning properly and in a good state of health.

The amount of energy provided by food is measured in calories or joules. The average man, assuming he is moderately active, needs

2,900 calories (12·1 MJ) and the average woman, because she is smaller, needs 2,200 calories (9·2 MJ) each day. Two-thirds of this energy is used just to keep the body alive, the heart beating, the lungs expanding and the liver and kidneys working. The rest is used for growth and activity.

The work of keeping the body ticking over is called the resting metabolism. Babies and young children have a faster metabolic rate than adults and therefore need proportionately more energy to meet their basic needs. Very fat people may make the excuse that they have a slower metabolic rate, but this is only true in exceptional cases. It is true, however, that they can become much more efficient at using as little energy as possible to do the same amount of work. This means they require even less energy in the form of food.

Energy can be obtained from all food whether it contains carbohydrate, fat, protein or alcohol, but the amount of energy provided by the different nutrients varies greatly:

1 gram fat   provides   9 Cal (37 Kilojoules)
1 gram alcohol   provides   7 Cal (29 K J)
1 gram protein   provides   4 Cal (17 K J)
1 gram carbohydrate provides 3·75 Cal (16 K J)

If the body cannot get enough energy from food then the stores of body fat are used. Conversely, if you eat more food than you need – no matter whether it be protein, fat or carbohydrate – it is converted into body fat and stored.

How Many Calories Do You Need?

Body weight only remains constant when your calorie intake matches your calorie expenditure. On the whole, less energy is used (less calories expended) as you become older and Appendixes 2 and 3, pages 294–5, give a good idea of the number of calories needed by a person at different life stages and engaged in various activities.

The more exercise taken the more energy is burned up. Even a brisk half-hour walk will use 100 calories more than just watching television for the same period. Apart from the obvious benefits, exercise also helps control your appetite. A little regular exercise has been shown to actually lower the appetites of sedentary workers. With intense exercise the appetite increases.

When reading Appendixes 2 and 3, it is important to remember that they are for the 'average' person. They might not apply to you at all. Everyone is different. Some people inherit a tendency to fatness, while others cannot put on weight however hard they try. It may seem unfair, but if you really do eat half as much as your skinny friend, and still put on weight, then you are eating too much and need to cut down.

Striking a Balance

As well as satisfying our energy requirements, food also provides the necessary nutrients for health. We need to take a closer look at these nutrients: protein, fat, carbohydrate, vitamins, minerals and water, in order to create a diet to suit ourselves. As nearly all foods are mixtures of nutrients, the wider the variety of foods eaten, the more likely it is that the essential nutrients will be provided.

Protein

Protein is necessary for growth and the renewal of body tissues, such as muscles, skin and blood, used in the process of living. Rich sources of protein are meat, fish, eggs, cheese and milk, and these animal protein foods provide the body with a whole range of amino acids, as well as vitamins and minerals, which can be used to build our tissues. Valuable proteins are also found in vegetable foods. The high protein content of soyabeans has been exploited to provide 'texturized vegetable protein' made to look and taste like meat. All pulses, such as baked beans, peas, beans and lentils provide protein. In fact 1 oz (28 g) lentils and 4 oz (113 g) baked beans contain as much protein as 1 oz (28 g) meat. Cereals and nuts are also useful sources of protein.

Fats

Fats are rich energy-giving foods, derived from plants and animals. Animal fats, like lard, suet and butter tend to be solid at room temperature, with the exception of the oils in fatty fish. Fats from plants, such as corn oil, sunflower and olive oil are liquid at room temperature. Some fat is necessary in our diet to provide essential fatty acids and the fat-soluble vitamins but whether liquid or solid 1 gram of pure fat provides 9 calories (27 KJ) and supplies a very concentrated source of energy.

All the animal protein foods mentioned earlier contain fat, and as these foods are digested more slowly and stay in the stomach longer they are sustaining and help to delay hunger pangs. However, without fully realizing it, our intake of fat may be unnecessarily high. Many baked, tinned or ready-made foods are hidden sources of fat. Fat increases the energy value of the diet without increasing the bulk, it also improves the palatability which encourages over-consumption. In other words you enjoy the food better when combined with fat and even when eating more than you need you do not fully realize that you have over-eaten.

Cholesterol is by now a familiar word to a lot of people. It is a natural fatty substance produced by the liver and transported in the bloodstream to other parts of the body where it is needed. Young babies need cholesterol for their brains to develop properly and adults need it for the formation of such vital substances as sex hormones.

There are two ways of obtaining cholesterol. It can either be made in the body by the liver, or it can be obtained from eggs, offal meats, and butter. However, the amount of cholesterol transported in the blood is influenced, not by dietary sources of cholesterol, but by the amount of saturated or hard fat in the diet. Saturated fat is found in most animal fats, cream cheese, butter and most margarines.

Some people have high levels of cholesterol and other fats in their bloodstream, which can build up and become deposited on the walls of the arteries. This happens especially if the arteries are damaged. Cholesterol plaques can build up and narrow the arteries, so that a blockage or clot occurs. Such a thrombosis can be the cause of a heart attack.

People with a high level of blood cholesterol carry a greater risk of developing coronary heart disease and it is advisable for such people to lower that risk by eating less saturated fat. We discuss the other important factors involved such as smoking, lack of exercise and tension under the section on heart attacks, page 220.

Carbohydrates

Carbohydrates are the sugars and starches, which provide the major source of food energy in our diets. Cellulose, although strictly a form of carbohydrate, cannot be utilized as a source of energy in man, but it does serve a vital function in providing roughage, or fibre (see page 79).

Ordinary table sugar (sucrose), glucose and syrups are the most concentrated sources of carbohydrate, but as they provide no other nutrients, are often referred to as giving 'empty calories'. Our preference for sweetness is pampered to in the form of cakes, pastries, biscuits, preserves and confectionery which are all too easy to eat to excess. A drastic reduction of such foods could not cause a lack of essential nutrients and would most certainly improve our health.

Sugar is also found in fruit and some vegetables but these foods supply vitamins and minerals in addition. They also contain a lot of water and cellulose which makes these foods useful 'fillers' and not 'fatteners'. Milk also provides sugar.

Starchy foods, such as cereals, grains, nuts, pulses and root vegetables are a valuable source of energy and also provide protein, some B vitamins and other nutrients.

Refined carbohydrates, such as polished white rice and white flour products, lose some of their nutrients during processing and in particular lose their fibrous, bulky layers, thus making them more concentrated and more easily over-consumed. Most breakfast cereals and all flour and bread sold in the U.K. are fortified with additional vitamins and some minerals although the amount of fibre may be limited.

Carbohydrates from unrefined, bulky cereals and pulses form an important part of any diet but sugar-intake should be restricted.

Vitamins

Vitamins are very important for our health and well-being. Only minute quantities of more than a dozen different vitamins are needed, but they are essential for growth and to enable the body to use other nutrients for energy. Vitamins help protect the body against infection and disease and generally aid the body to work efficiently.

Vitamin A is needed in order to see in dim light and to maintain the health of the skin and mucous membranes. It is essential for normal growth and development. It is virtually impossible to go short of this vitamin, as it is found in so many foods. The richest sources of vitamin A are liver, kidney, the fish liver oils, and also margarine, eggs and dairy products; milk and cream contain slightly more in summer than in winter. Oily fish, other offal, molluscs (like mussels) also contain small amounts. Carrots and other dark green and yellow vegetables and fruits contain the orange-yellow pigment carotene which is converted into vitamin A by the body.

The B group of vitamins are required for healthy growth and in particular for the release of energy from food. They are essential for the metabolism of nerve tissue and are necessary for the formation of new blood cells.

Several different B vitamins are known, but many of them are found together in foods like meat, particularly offal meats like liver, kidneys, and heart; eggs, some dairy produce and cereal foods, especially products made from enriched refined cereals and wholegrains.

Vitamin C is essential to keep tissues healthy and help wounds to heal. It also aids the absorption of iron from our food.

Vitamin C is found mainly in citrus and berry fruits, in green vegetables, salads and potatoes. Unfortunately, although most fresh fruits and vegetables contain some vitamin C this may be lost during storage, preparation and cooking. Unlike vitamins A and D, vitamin C cannot be stored by the body and a lack of it causes sluggishness, slow wound-healing and bleeding from small blood vessels. It is more likely to be an orange rather than an apple which keeps the doctor away.

Smoking may increase the need for vitamin C. Smoking is a hazard to your health in many ways, but if you really cannot give it up, you should take care to include more foods containing this vitamin in your daily diet.

Vitamin D is often called the 'sunshine' vitamin for although it is partly derived from food, it is also manufactured in the body itself when sunlight falls on the skin. It is necessary for the deposition of calcium and phosphorus in bones and is particularly important during periods of growth. Without it, rickets can occur.

Food sources of vitamin D are fish-liver oils, fatty fish, such as herrings, mackerel, salmon and sardines, margarine and eggs. Dairy foods (butter, milk and cheese) and liver contain small quantities.

Vitamin E is widely distributed in our food, the richest source being vegetable oil, especially wheatgerm oil. It is also found in green and other vegetables and in nuts and some fruits.

Unfortunately, contrary to popular claim, extra vitamin E does not help problems such as infertility or baldness. The only deficiency that has ever been demonstrated in man is in premature babies who are bottle fed.

Vitamin pills are really unnecessary for most people who are eating a varied diet. However, when there are extra demands, such as during pregnancy and breast feeding, extra vitamins and minerals are advisable. Added vitamins can also help after an operation or severe illness.

All children up to two years old should take vitamins A, C, and D while their food intake is still small. Extra vitamins can be useful during convalescence after an illness or operation and possibly in old age.

Children living in high-rise flats and people who are unable to go out may well need added vitamin D, as the lack of sunshine can lead to a deficiency. Vitamins can be toxic if taken in excess and no amount of vitamin pills can turn a bad diet into a good one!

Minerals

A well-balanced diet must include small quantities of minerals. Altogether many different minerals are needed for health. Most of these are widely distributed in foods. Some care needs to be taken to obtain adequate iron and calcium, but it is unlikely that other minerals will be lacking.

Iron is needed for the production of the red blood cells which take oxygen round the body. Iron-deficiency anaemia makes oxygen transportation inefficient, and this results in fatigue, depression and a general slowing down of most body processes.

Main sources of this mineral are offal and red meat, eggs, bread, flour, and oatmeal. Small amounts of iron are in dried fruit and cocoa, but not, as popularly thought, in dark green vegetables like spinach and watercress. However, it is the vitamin C in these vegetables that improves the absorption of iron during digestion.

Calcium builds healthy bones and teeth in conjunction with vitamin D, and it is needed for the contraction of muscles and for good nerve function. Milk and cheese are good sources, and the soft edible bones in canned fish, such as salmon and sardines are useful too. In the U.K. most flour products are fortified with calcium and 'hard' water contains significant amounts of calcium.

Salt is needed to maintain the concentration of body fluids and occurs naturally in many types of food. The average diet contains four or five times more than the amount strictly needed, because of the amount which is added in cooking. Most of us would do well to restrict our intake.

Fibre

Fibre, until recently, has been the 'forgotten factor' in our food. Roughage, or 'dietary fibre' is found in the outer husk of cereal grains, in fruit, and in the leaves, stems and roots of vegetables. This indigestible material is essential to provide the bulk which absorbs water and takes the waste products through the body.

Many diseases of the colon and bowel have been attributed to the 'low-fibre' diet preferred in modern industrialized countries. Bran, the husk of the wheatgrain, is by far the best laxative for the prevention of constipation. Doctors recommend that everyone should increase their fibre intake by including unrefined foods in their diet, such as wholegrain cereals, in addition to fruit and a generous supply of vegetables.

Failing this, natural bran can be taken every day. Additional bran is helpful to the elderly who are housebound and inactive, and also to slimmers, as it adds to the feeling of fullness in the stomach.

Water

The greatest part of the body is water, and although we could last for quite a long time without food, we cannot survive for long without water. Most adults drink about 3 pints (1·7 l) of fluid a day and derive a further 2 pints (1·1 l) or so from their food. The kidneys keep a very fine control of the concentration of body fluids. Except in certain medical conditions, there is no need to limit the daily intake of fluid, indeed it is important to drink more fluid rather than too little. Too little can lead to constipation or to dehydration, particularly in elderly people who are worried about getting up in the night.

Water taken in excess of requirements is simply excreted by the kidneys as urine. Water is also lost by sweating and from the lungs and in the faeces. Never restrict the water intake even when slimming, provided the fluids consumed do not contain sugar and exceed the daily calorie allowance. It is too often forgotten that milk is a food!

Eating to Suit Yourself

In thinking of Slimnastics as a way of life, the aim for each of us is to create a balanced nutritious eating pattern so that we not only remain healthy but also really enjoy living! However, we eat for many other reasons than simply to stay alive; it gives us pleasure and forms the focus of so many social events. It is so much part of our daily lives, that changing our habits is not always easy.

It would be foolish therefore to pretend that cutting down on food intake in order to lose weight or even rethinking our eating habits, is not going to be hard work, especially at the beginning. This is where the Slimnastics group can offer such good moral support and encouragement. It is a much more difficult task to carry out alone.

The first step is to find out exactly how you are eating at the moment. For one week write down *every single thing* you eat and drink each day. Either fill in the Diet Sheet (see Appendix 7) or make one of your own (it might have to be slightly larger!). It will probably be a revelation to you. If you do need to lose weight you may well have lost some by the end of the week – who is going to admit, even to themselves, to the second Mars Bar or third whisky!

If you are eating a nutritious, balanced diet, your sheet will show:

PROTEIN every day (preferably a mixture of animal and vegetable proteins and maybe textured vegetable protein).

Some CARBOHYDRATE every day in the form of wholemeal bread, pulses, pasta, rice or potato.

Sufficient vegetables and fruit to provide VITAMINS, MINERALS and FIBRE.

Enough FLUID every day.

We all need to cut down the fats in our diet – we must look carefully at how our food is cooked; the convenience foods we eat and also the dressings we put on salads. We can all do without the pure carbohydrate of sugar.

The next step is to weigh yourself – if possible on scales which have been checked by the Weights and Measures Board, such as those at the local chemist or at the doctor's surgery.

Having weighed yourself, study the Ideal-weight Charts (see Appendix 5) and, making allowance for your bone structure, find the weight you ought to be. If you discover that you are either under or are average weight according to these charts you should nevertheless still complete a diet sheet to check that you are eating well. You might still have too much fat and not enough muscle. As you tone up your muscles with exercise and they increase in weight, you may well have to cut down your food intake in order to compensate.

If you are more than 10 per cent over your average weight, you need to slim. The way you tackle this depends very much on you – the sort of person you are, the life you are leading and the mistakes you are making. Do not be put off by the thought that you will not be able to eat so well. So many people resist any form of slimming in the fear that it will spoil their enjoyment of life, 'We have only one life, let's live it to the full,' they say! Let us do just that, but at the same time grasp the truth that it is perfectly possible to eat excellently and yet be healthy. We need to eat well but wisely!

We need to discuss the different approaches you can take to this problem and then we will think of ways you can help yourself.

Some Different Approaches to the Weight Problem

Counting* calories

Whatever you eat, whether it is lettuce, celery, steak, white fish or caviare, bread, potatoes or cream cakes, contains calories, though in different amounts. Slimmers need calories like everyone else but they

---

*A calorie is the expression of energy contained in food and drink, and one calorie is a very small unit. Normally food energy is measured in kilocalories. In the text a calorie is taken to mean a kilocalorie (usually designated a Calorie, with a capital C) and is equivalent to 1,000 calories.

should have fewer of them. The actual number of calories any one person needs is almost impossible to determine outside a hospital metabolic unit. Individuals vary in their energy requirements. *What we can say, however, is that the daily intake of calories should always match the daily expenditure of energy.*

Given normal conditions, if you are gaining weight, however slowly, you have been generally exceeding your calorie requirement. If your body weight stays steady for months on end, you can tell that you are eating exactly the right number of calories to suit your own, highly personal, energy needs.

If you are prepared to weigh everything you eat, you can find out approximately how many calories you are consuming from the Food-for-fitness Calorie Tables, pages 94–102, in this book. (Do not forget to include such items as the knob of butter in the mashed potatoes, the spoonful of sugar on the grapefruit!)

Low-carbohydrate diet

Since a 'low-carbohydrate' diet means that you will be cutting out the 'sweet sticky stodge' (the biscuits, cream buns, steamed jam puddings, cakes, etc.) it is in effect a calorie-controlled diet as these foods contain a lot of fat too. But – and it is a big But – you must remember that many high-protein foods such as pork, ham, bacon, eggs and cheese are also very high in energy-giving fat and therefore their calorie content is very high too. You must be careful not to eat an excessive amount of these foods.

Many people can successfully lose weight merely by restricting the carbohydrate content of their diet. They do not have to count calories, only the carbohydrate units, eating as far as possible only high-protein foods and low-calorie fruits and vegetables. On this diet you need to beware of 'made-up' goods and to check the ingredients when you buy convenience foods. (The label has to show all the ingredients in decreasing order of quantity.) However, the low-carbohydrate diet is deficient in bran needed to prevent constipation which is common in slimmers. The fibre from bread and potatoes is helpful in preventing this, while that from fruit and vegetables is less efficient.

Cutting down the fat

Cutting down (which is not the same as cutting out) the fat will greatly reduce the calories in the diet of any normal adult or child as fat provides twice as many calories as protein or carbohydrate.

There are a number of ways to reduce the fat you eat. Use recipes which require less fat (we show you how to adapt recipes in the cookery section); always grill rather than fry and use non-stick pans as these need little or no fat for cooking. Remember that soft margarine and oils provide just as many calories as the other fats. You must cut down on these. Pickle or tomato will often substitute on your bread or sandwiches for providing extra moisture. Eat more foods like chicken, fish, fruits, vegetables and cereal grains as an alternative to meat, eggs and cheese. The meats shown with the highest calorie content in the Food-for-fitness Calorie Tables (see pages 94–102) are those that contain most fat. Avoid these as much as you can. Also try to avoid made-up convenience foods which are high in hidden fat.

Crash diets

These are a quick way of losing the few odd pounds but are no good in the long run and can be dangerous. If you slim hard for a while, then stop and then start again you upset your metabolism and make it all the more difficult to adjust. The same applies to some of the 'gimmick' diets you read in magazines. Naturally if the total calories of the recommended diet add up to less than those you are already eating you will undoubtedly lose weight but as the diet recommended is usually not your natural way of eating you will soon revert to your bad old ways and your weight will gradually creep up again.

Health farms and clinics

Oh, the luxury of being told what to do, of being pampered and cared for; the lovely idea of handing over the discipline and self-control to someone else! It will cost a lot of money and you will probably have a much earned rest but it is unlikely to work as a long-term weight cure. Once you are back in your own surroundings and having to rely on your own determination – ten to one you will go back to your old habits! Of course they will be only too glad to welcome you back again – and again . . .!

'Slimming foods'

When the advertisements say 'slimming' they mean 'less fattening' though in many cases the advertised 'slimmers' meals' such as puddings, soups, sweets and bread are often no lower in energy than normal foods, weight for weight, and are of limited value in controlling the weight in the long term unless part of a calorie-controlled diet (by law this has to be written on the packet). It is much better to establish good eating patterns with normal food than with substitutes. If you forget your sweeteners for a tea party – you will take the sugar offered, your crispbread too is probably coated with butter and jam!

'Old wives' tales'

Acids such as grapefruit, lemon juice or vinegar are sometimes claimed to 'burn up fat'. This is a fallacy. If these substances do help to reduce weight it is due to their effect of aiding some people to overcome a sweet tooth. However an unsweetened grapefruit can act as a very useful filler or as a low-calorie starter to a meal.

Other diets restrict salt and fluid, causing a loss of weight but no loss of fat. Except when medically advised, there is no need to exclude salt, and water should never be restricted. On the contrary, if you drink water with your meals it can help you by giving a feeling of fullness.

How About You?

Now that we have got the theories straightened out and in perspective, how are *you* going to lose weight? One thing is clear – to lose weight you must cut down on your calorie intake. To do this you could count calories, but calorie counting is often impractical, certainly for any length of time (you would need to consult your calorie chart at every meal you eat!) and counting calories may lead to an

unbalanced diet. You could reduce carbohydrate foods and concentrate on high-protein foods (*but* many of these are high in calories),
or you could cut down the fat in your diet. A far better way to lose
weight is to combine cutting down on the fat with cutting out the
unnecessary carbohydrate foods – the refined cereals and the refined
starches (meaning *no* white flour and *no* added sugar at all, including
sugar in any of its disguises such as biscuits, cakes, pastries, etc.!).

Certainly, by a reduction in fat and omission of refined starches
from your daily diet, you should lose weight, but that will not be the
only benefit. As we have seen, too much fat in our diet is actively
bad for us. So too is the lack of roughage; but we can all do without
any refined starches and sugars as they add little but calories to a
well-balanced diet. This means that *everyone* will benefit by following
these principles. In the next chapter we give you The Golden Rules
for Healthy Cooking. Follow these and you will create an eating
pattern and content which is good for both 'body and soul'!

It is not only important that you should understand food, its basic
constituents and its effect on the body, and also weight control and
how it can be achieved, it is also essential to understand the particular
problems associated with eating and the mistakes which you may
have been making. When you fully recognize your 'addictions',
transgressions and/or follies, or even perhaps a medical cause, you
will be better able to put the principles of healthy eating into practice. To do this we need to look at your diet sheet again and ask a few
questions.

Are you eating at regular intervals?

Remember that it is a regularly stoked fire which retains its heat and
burns best. If we think of food as fuel for our boiler it makes sense
that we should feed it properly at regular intervals. There are members of our Slimnastics groups who have lost weight simply by
beginning to eat more protein-rich foods and less carbohydrate-rich
foods for breakfast. This helps them to resist the temptation of the
mid-morning snack and gives them more long-term energy to work
better. All teachers will recognize the drooping under-achieving
child who has not had breakfast. If food first thing is impossible to
face, either get up a little earlier or eat it as soon as you can, even if
this does mean taking some food to work or eating it after the

children have gone to school. This applies to other meals too. It may suit us to eat our main meal mid-day or in the evening but either way we should not skip the other meals.

Are you a 'sweetness addict'?

Is your diet sheet full of such goodies as buns, biscuits, sweets and puddings? Some people develop a real craving for sugar and find these foods very difficult to give up. It takes strong willpower but you can eventually re-educate your sense of taste. Six weeks without sugar in your tea and coffee and you will not like it either way! But persevere, six more weeks and you will never have sugar in it again. You will have begun to appreciate the taste of the drink itself.

Some people find it easier to give up all sweet foods entirely, others have to take it more gradually – first banning sweet foods before lunch-time, then extending this to tea time, etc. Others find it essential to leave enough calories over each day for a moderate quantity of these 'sinful luxuries'. It is like giving up smoking – if one way does not succeed you must try another. A good compromise is to allow one day a week off to indulge yourself a little. Gradually your appetite will shrink as you lose weight and your taste will change and soon this day of indulgence will become less sinful too!

Are you a fat fanatic?

Perhaps you think of yourself as a person who is eating a good high-protein diet. However, check your written chart very carefully. It may be full of extra calories; the butter with the beans, the fat to fry the liver, the cream on the fruit, the oil in the salad dressing, the olives in the stew. Look at the Calorie Tables (see pages 94–102) and see how high in calories are many of the meats, cheese and dairy foods. One of the most common mistakes amongst the members of our Slimnastics groups is to misjudge the quantity of cheese they are eating – the chunk they cut themselves for a quick reviving snack may well equal the calories eaten for a whole meal! The cheese and biscuits idled over at the end of a carefully balanced dinner may add up to more calories than the rest of the food put together. Nuts too are very 'moreish'.

Check the contents on tins and of convenience foods on the delicatessen counter, many of them are very high in fat content. Fat is not mentioned on tinned-meat products but it is present all the same – beware!

As we have said before, cutting down on the refined cereals and sugars will automatically decrease your fat intake. Learn to cook with the minimum of fat – use our cookery chapter and cook delicious meals.

Are you an alcoholic?

We do not mean this literally but we do mean, 'Are you drinking too much alcohol?' Drinking in moderation can be a source of pleasure and comfort, beneficial both to our social welfare and to our health. Unfortunately, we have noticed over the past few years a marked increase in the amounts consumed and dependence on alcohol in all age groups from 18 to old age, with its consequent effects not only on weight but also health, with sometimes degrading or even tragic results. Drinking without control is beyond our brief and needs professional help. Casually drinking to excess though is another matter and to achieve fitness and health without excess weight alcohol needs to be cut down to a moderate amount.

Alcohol is a rich source of calories quickly absorbed by the body. If you dance at a disco until the early hours – an energetic and enjoyable way of burning up calories – and you are also drinking alcohol, you will be using that alcohol as the energy to keep your body going and you will be retaining the fat you might have lost! Not only that, you will probably have retained the calories from the alcoholic drink itself (see the Calorie Tables pages 94–102) so that, when you have regained the fluid lost in perspiration, you might find that you have actually gained weight. Not only does alcohol retain your weight, it also depresses the nervous system and releases the inhibitions. This is when the over-eating and drinking can begin!

Slimmers do not want to feel anti-social, but there are plenty of ways you can cut down without actually advertising the fact that you are taking care. For a start choose a drink which is lowest in calories and make use of the low-calorie tonics and bitter lemons, etc. Fizzy drinks are absorbed more quickly into the bloodstream so even a limited amount of alcohol plus fizz will give you a 'lift'. Drink more slowly and when refilling your glass do so from the soda bottle. The empty glass is the one which is replenished. *Never* drink alone and preferably only with food.

Are you eating for a former life?

Time and again we hear the woeful cry, 'I cannot understand it – I've always eaten like this and have only just begun to put on weight.' It may be that you are still eating the correct amount for an active young person though you are in fact just beginning to settle into a sedentary middle age! Our metabolic rate does change especially at different 'life stages'. We have given more individual help on this in Chapter 8, page 185.

Are you an unconscious nibbler?

You may be eating very well balanced meals but inbetween times unthinkingly consuming almost as many calories again. Biscuits with coffee, sweets in the car, nuts and chocolates in front of T.V., ice creams at the cinema; you can eat them without even registering that these snacks are *food*. You will still be quite ready for the following meal. Good cooks have their problems too – a taste here, a lick there, a bowl to clean, one spoonful left over – all these can disappear and not be noticed.

Busy people too can eat hundreds of calories and still feel that they are due for a meal. Think of the busy mother with a part-time job, feeding the family well for breakfast but not leaving much time for herself, just grabbing at the easiest things like cereal and toast plus the children's leftovers, the crusts of toast, the rind of the bacon; off to work, she has a mid-morning low and so has sugar and a biscuit with her coffee; rushing home at lunch-time she eats 'on the trot' a piece of cheese, an apple and leftovers, another sliver of cheese, a choc bar 'to give her a lift', another bite of cheese, etc.; she rushes around with housework; she picks the children up, collapses into a chair when she feeds them tea and has a piece of cake (after all she has missed lunch!); then perhaps has a drink in the evening with her husband after a very busy day and before the evening meal. She cannot think why she puts on weight – she is a very busy person always on the go and often 'missing' meals. The same effect can be felt by the man who travels for a living – it is a busy life but snack meals in the car add up to lots of calories and little in the way of exercise.

Try to make every mouthful an occasion. It is not only the snacks that disappear without notice. If you eat your meal very fast while you are talking or watching television you can empty your plate almost before you register its contents and then you will be asking for more. The same will happen if you finish your plateful before the others at the table. Take your time to eat, savour all the tastes. If you encourage yourself to appreciate all you eat you will consume less but end up more satisfied.

Are you eating too much?

If none of the above applies to you and you are eating nutritious food but are still overweight your calorie input has exceeded your calorie output. If this is so, you must actually make the effort to count the calories you are eating. Weigh out the food you eat for a normal day and add up the calories (see the Calorie Tables, pages 94–102). Be careful not to underestimate; do not forget the crisps eaten at the cinema or the rich sauce you had at a dinner party.

When you have added up your total calorie intake for a day (or preferably a week) you will have to lower your intake and also increase your output by more exercise in order to burn up excess fat. Be careful to include in your diet all the essential nutrients. To help you do this we have asked one of our consultant dieticians to compile an easy-to-follow nutritious low-sugar restricted-fat diet (see pages 92–4). This is for approximately 1,200 calories a day. Remember that this calorie level may be too high or too low for you and you should adapt it accordingly. No one should go on a diet of less than 1,000 a day without medical approval.

This diet should only be used by those who really need it. Alongside the dieticians, we feel that calorie counting is often impractical and can become a phobia. It would be much better for you to work out a balanced diet to suit yourself, cutting out the unnecessary foods and avoiding the high-carbohydrate/high-fat foods.

Is exercise your answer?

Exercise alone is not sufficient to lose weight; in fact as we have seen you may gain slightly through the regained muscle tone which weighs more than the fat lost. However, some people, especially athletes, sportsmen and women, gymnasts, ballet dancers and the like – find it very difficult indeed to lose excess weight by diet alone. They really do seem to need to increase their energy output more than those who have led more inactive lives. These are the people who will particularly benefit by exercising regularly and taking up such calorie-burners as swimming and jogging.

Are you affected by social pressures?

It is not only important to find out how you are burdening yourself with this extra weight but also the reasons why you are eating in this way. After all, it is no use working hard to put ourselves to rights if we have not sought out the root of the problem.

Many pressures induce a person to eat – we eat because food is available; we eat because we need a break; we eat to unwind; we eat out of frustration and boredom. Without the social ties of family and friends, many people who are on their own all day, such as the elderly and young mothers, never bother to make themselves meals but nibble constantly all day long. We eat for comfort – if we dislike our job or home life is unhappy, eating can be a solace. Maybe we have just followed our family traditions, fat families can breed fat families! Remember that many people over-eat for these reasons but only some put on weight. Those are the ones who are unfortunately adding to their difficulties and must make every effort to seek a solution to the problem.

When should you seek medical help?

You might well be sent away with a 'flea in your ear' if you go to your G.P. complaining that your clothes do not fit, you do not like yourself in a bikini or you have not lost your excess weight after your last baby/hysterectomy, etc.! You will receive much more attention if, having tried all the above suggestions, you then consult your doctor and mention any side-effects such as breathlessness, tiredness, aches and pains in the joints, swollen ankles, etc. When he recommends going on a diet, you can then say you have been trying and show him four weeks of completed diet sheets together with a weight check. Doctors are more inclined to believe facts than a garbled story. There are some medical conditions which do contribute to excess weight and your doctor will consider them seriously provided he knows that you have explored all other avenues first.

You also need to take into account any medication you are already taking. The oral contraceptive can cause weight gain, but so do steroids, some anti-depressants, some tranquillizers, and some anti-inflammatory drugs. Ask the chemist if your medicine can have side-effects of this kind. *Do not stop taking them* unless you ask your doctor. Remember that as soon as you are able to cease taking them, your weight will probably return to normal.

Women can gain weight through fluid retention prior to their period. This can result in unpleasant premenstrual tension and we discuss this fully on pages 187–90.

Giving up smoking tends to contribute to weight gain but this usually settles down after six months. Sometimes the extra weight is due to the substitution of sweets for cigarettes or to an increased desire for food because of undulled taste buds. It will certainly pay in this case to watch calorie intakes and perhaps recent non-smokers should make every effort to exercise more. They will have more breath to do so!

Wishing will get you nowhere!

Unfortunately, like the child who longs to wake up in the morning speaking fluent French, we cannot just *wish* to lose weight. Nor, for the child, does it matter how good his French teachers are, he still has to do all the work himself; the teacher can encourage, cajole, inspire but ultimately the work has to be done by the child himself. It is just the same with slimming. Only *you* can achieve the desired results and no one else can be in charge – not your family, friends or even your doctor.

We hope that we have encouraged you to create for yourself a new approach to your eating as well as a well-balanced nutritional diet.

Now to action!

1. Learn the facts about the food you have been eating and the food you should be eating.
2. Write out your diet sheet. It is impossible to help yourself if you just guess what you are eating and drinking day by day.
3. Check your diet sheet for quality and quantity and also for the mistakes that you are making. Study the ways to control your weight.
4. Decide on the eating pattern with a good nutritional content which suits you and your way of living – The Food-for-fitness Eating Guide and The Food-for-fitness Calorie Tables together with carbohydrate units are on pages 92–102.
5. Read the next chapter Cooking and Eating for Fitness – this shows you how to take action and enjoy it!

It will be worth it – a healthy balanced diet is an essential foundation stone when building a fit way of life.

The Food-for-fitness Eating Guide

Use this guide in conjunction with The Food-for-fitness Calorie Tables (see pages 94–102). Check each food for approximate calories and carbohydrate units. The more weight you have to lose the more you should concentrate on low-calorie foods in each category. This nutritious low-sugar restricted-fat diet has been compiled by one of our consultant dieticians and is for approximately 1,200 calories a day.

Eat:

Three meals a day (with no nibbling in between!). Every meal should include a food chosen from each of the following three categories:

CATEGORY 1

Base each meal on *one* of the following protein-containing foods:
Lean meat, poultry, offal.
White or oily fish (drained of oil).

Cheese – use in moderation and check the calories (no cream cheese).
Eggs.
2 tablespoons pulse vegetables (peas, beans or lentils).

CATEGORY 2

Include just *one* of these starch foods at each meal:
1 small slice bread (any variety).
1 cup breakfast cereal (unsweetened).
2 crispbreads (wheat or rye).
1 small potato (you can eat the skin too).
1 tablespoon rice (white or brown).
1 carton natural yogurt.

CATEGORY 3

Always include leafy vegetables, salads or small servings of root vegetables.

In addition:

Have 1 or 2 portions of fruit a day.
Include ½ pint (284 ml) milk for use in tea or coffee.
Drink as much water, sugar-free drinks, meat extract or bouillon as you like.

Avoid:

(*a*) Absolutely everything containing sugar. This includes all confectionery, sweets, chocolate, sugars, glucose, honey, syrup, treacle, preserves.
(*b*) Drinks such as cordials, fizzy drinks and fruit squash.

Check:

The ingredients of 'made-up' products and avoid those containing sugar, fat and starch. This includes sugared breakfast cereals, creamed, thickened, tinned and packet soups, baked goods and puddings, including biscuits, cakes, buns, scones, pies, pastries, batter mixtures, milk puddings, mousse, ice cream, flavoured yogurt, sweetened tinned fruit.

Restrict:

Your use of butter, margarine, salad oils and cooking fats. Never fry and avoid all fatty meats, mayonnaise and sauces made with cheese, oil or any other fat.

Limit:

Your alcohol intake, especially beer, ale, stout and cider. One small dry drink is equivalent to one of the starchy foods (see Category 2).

The Food-for-fitness Calorie Tables

Unless otherwise stated these calories are for portions of 1 oz (28 g).
    When first using these lists weigh the foods you choose until you are able to judge fairly accurately the amounts you are using (some foods such as cheese can be misleading).
    At each meal include one food from Category 1, 2 and 3.

Table 1: *under 100 Calories*
(C.U. = Carbohydrate Units)

Category			Approx. Calories	C.U.
	DAIRY FOODS			
1	Bacon	– collar	70	0
1		gammon	100	0
1	Cheese	– Camembert	90	0
1		Cottage	30	0
1		Curd	40	0
1		Edam	90	0
1		Gouda	100	0
1		smoked	80	0
1	Eggs		50	0
	Milk	– ½ pint (284 ml) (skimmed)	100	2½
2	Yogurt	– flavoured	30	0
		low-fat	20	0

Table 1: under 100 Calories—continued

Category			Approx. Calories	C.U.
	FISH			
1	Anchovies		40	0
1	Bloaters		80	0
1	Clams		20	0
1	Cockles		20	0
1	Cod		20	0
1	Crab		40	0
1	Eels (smoked)		50	0
1	Flounder		20	0
1	Haddock		20	0
1	Halibut		30	0
1	Herring		70	0
1	Kippers		30	0
1	Lobster		20	0
1	Mussels		10	0
1	Octopus		30	0
1	Oysters		10	0
1	Perch		40	0
1	Pike		30	0
1	Pilchards		60	0
1	Plaice		20	0
1	Pollack		30	0
1	Prawns		30	0
1	Roe	– Cod	40	0
		Herring	80	0
1	Salmon	– canned	40	0
		raw	60	0
1	Sardines	– canned in oil	100	0
1	Scallop		30	0
1	Skate		30	0
1	Sole		30	0
1	Squid		30	0
1	Sturgeon		30	0
1	Trout		30	0
1	Tuna	– canned in oil	90	0
1	Whelks		30	0
1	Whiting		20	0
	FRUIT			
	Apples		10	½

Table 1: under 100 Calories—continued

Category			Approx. Calories	C.U.
Apricots	– dried		60	½
	fresh		10	½
Avocado			50	Neg
Banana			30	1
Blackberries			10	½
Blackcurrants			10	½
Cherries			20	½
Clementines			20	½
Cranberries			10	½
Currants	– dried		70	3½
Damsons			10	½
Dates	– dried		80	4
	fresh		40	½
Ginger	– ground		80	3½
Gooseberries	– cooking		10	½
	dessert		10	½
Greengages			20	1
Grapefruit			10	Neg
Grapes	– black		20	1
	white		20	1
Figs	– dried		70	3
	fresh		20	1
Lemon			10	Neg
Lemon juice			10	Neg
Loganberries			20	1
Mandarines			20	1
Melons	– canteloupe		10	Neg
	honeydew		10	Neg
	Ogen		10	Neg
	yellow		10	Neg
Mulberries			10	½
Nectarines			20	1
Olives			30	Neg
Oranges			10	½
Palm fruit			60	2½
Passion fruit			10	1
Peaches			20	½
Pears			10	½
Pineapple			20	1

Table 1: under 100 Calories—continued

Category			Approx. Calories	C.U.
	Plums		10	½
	Prunes		40	1
	Pomegranate		20	1
	Pumpkin		10	Neg
	Quinces		10	½
	Raisin		70	4
	Raspberries		10	½
	Redcurrants		10	Neg
	Rhubarb		10	Neg
	Satsumas		20	1
	Strawberries		10	½
	Sultanas		80	4
	Tangerines		20	1
	Tomatoes		10	½
	Water melons		10	½
	MEAT			
1	Beef	– brisket	70	0
1		lean steak	40	0
1		mince	70	0
1		silverside	70	0
1		sirloin (lean)	70	0
1		stewing steak	80	0
1		topside	80	0
1	Chicken	– no skin	40	0
1	Duck	– no skin	40	0
1	Goose		60	0
1	Guinea fowl		60	0
1	Grouse		50	0
1	Ham	– lean	70	0
1	Lamb	– leg	90	0
1		shoulder	100	0
1		stewing	60	0
1	Mutton		90	0
1	Partridge		60	0
1	Pheasant		60	0
1	Pigeon		70	0
1	Pork	– leg	80	0
1		loin	100	0
1	Rabbit		40	0

N.P.S.—7

Table 1: under 100 Calories—continued

Category			Approx. Calories	C.U
1	Sausages	– beef (raw)	90	1
1	Turkey		40	0
1	Veal		40	0
1	Venison		60	0
	OFFAL			
1	Heart		50	0
1	Kidney		30	0
1	Liver		70	0
1	Sweetbreads		30	0
1	Tongue	– ox (boiled)	90	0
		sheep (stewed)	90	0
1	Tripe		20	0
	VEGETABLES			
3	Artichokes	– globe	10	Neg
3		Jerusalem	10	Neg
3	Asparagus		10	Neg
3	Aubergines		10	Neg
1	Beans	– baked	30	1
1		broad	10	$\frac{1}{2}$
1		butter	30	1
1		haricot	80	1
1		kidney	80	1
3		runner	10	Neg
3	Bamboo shoots		10	$\frac{1}{2}$
3	Bean shoots		10	$\frac{1}{2}$
3	Beetroot		10	$\frac{1}{2}$
3	Broccoli		10	Neg
3	Brussels sprouts		10	Neg
3	Cabbage Red/White/Chinese		10	Neg
3	Calabrese		10	Neg
3	Carrots		10	$\frac{1}{2}$
3	Cauliflower		10	Neg
3	Celery		10	Neg
3	Celeriac		10	Neg
3	Chicory		10	Neg
3	Chillies		90	Neg
3	Chives		10	Neg
3	Courgettes		10	Neg

Table 1: under 100 Calories—continued

Category			Approx. Calories	C.U.
3	Cucumber		10	Neg
3	Endive		10	Neg
3	Fennel		10	Neg
3	Horseradish		40	1
3	Leeks		10	½
2	Lentils		90	3
3	Lettuce		10	Neg
3	Mangetout		10	Neg
3	Marrow		10	Neg
3	Mushrooms		10	Neg
3	Mustard and cress		10	Neg
3	Onions		10	Neg
3	Parsnips		10	½
1	Peas	– dried	90	3
3		fresh	20	1
1		split	90	3
3	Peppers		10	Neg
2	Potatoes		30	1
3	Pumpkin		10	Neg
3	Radish		10	Neg
3	Rhubarb		10	Neg
3	Salsify		10	Neg
3	Seakale		10	Neg
3	Spinach		10	Neg
3	Spring greens		10	Neg
3	Spring onions		10	Neg
3	Swede		10	½
3	Sweet corn		40	½
3	Turnips		10	½
3	Watercress		10	Neg
2	Water chestnuts		30	½
	CEREALS			
2	Bread	– brown	70	2½
2		hi bran	70	2½
2		starch reduced	70	1½
2		wheatgerm	70	2½
2		white	70	3
2		wholemeal	70	2½

Table 1: under 100 Calories—continued

Category			Approx. Calories	C.U.
2	Breakfast Cereals	– bran (1 tablespoon = 10 cal)	60	1½
2		flaked wheat	100	4½
2		puffed wheat	100	4
2		shredded wheat	100	5
2		wheatgerm	100	3
2		wholewheat	100	4
2	Cornflour		100	5
2	Flour	– brown	100	4½
2		white	100	4½
2		wholemeal	100	4

Table 2: under 200 Calories

Category		Approx. Calories	C.U.
	DAIRY FOODS		
1	Bacon – back (raw)	130	0
1	streaky (raw)	120	0
1	Cheese – Cheddar	120	0
1	Cheshire	110	0
1	Danish blue	110	0
1	Gruyère	130	0
1	Leicester	110	0
1	Parmesan	120	0
1	Stilton	140	0
1	Wensleydale	120	0
1	Milk – ½ pint (284 ml)	190	2½
	CEREALS		
2	Barley	110	4½
2	Pasta	110	4–5
2	Rice	110	5
2	Sago	110	5½
2	Semolina	110	4½
2	Soya flour	130	1½
	FISH		
1	Eels – fresh	110	0
	MEAT		
1	Pork sausage (grilled)	110	1
	NUTS AND SEEDS		
1	Almonds	170	Neg
1	Beechnuts	170	1
1	Brazil nuts	180	Neg
1	Cashew nuts	180	1½
1	Coconut – fresh	110	Neg
1	desiccated	180	Neg
1	Peanuts	170	½
1	Pistachio	180	1
1	Sesame seeds	170	1
1	Sunflower seeds	170	½
1	Walnuts	160	½
	VEGETABLES		
1	Soya beans	110	1½

Table 3: Calories—Liquids
(An approximation has been made for carbohydrate units: 1 g alcohol = 1·75 g carbohydrate – hence C.U. value for spirits.)

			Approx. Calories	C.U.
ALCOHOL				
Beer	– draught bitter	1 pint (570 ml)	180	9½
	draught mild	1 pint (570 ml)	140	7
	pale ale	1 pint (570 ml)	180	7½
	lager	1 pint (570 ml)	150	7½
	brown ale	1 pint (570 ml)	160	8½
	bottle stout	1 pint (570 ml)	200	12
Brandy		liqueur glass	75	3–4½
Bourbon		liqueur glass	65	2–4½
Cider	– dry	1 pint (570 ml)	200	10
	sweet	1 pint (570 ml)	240	20½
Gin		1 measure	55	3–4½
Liqueurs		vary according to type	115–300	3–4½
Port		1 measure	75	2–4½
Rum		1 measure	75	3–4½
Sherry	– dry	1 measure	55	1½
	sweet	1 measure	65	2
Vermouth	– dry	1 measure	55	1½
	sweet	1 measure	75	3½
Vodka		1 measure	65	3
Whisky		1 measure	60	3½
Wine	– dry	¼ pint (140 ml)	90	1–3
	sweet	¼ pint (140 ml)	115	1–5
SOFT DRINKS				
Apple juice, unsweetened, small glass			50	2½
Blackcurrant concentrate, 1 tablespoon			35	3½
Grapefruit juice, unsweetened, small glass			55	11½
Lemonade, 1 pint (570 ml)			120	2½
Orange juice, unsweetened, small glass			60	11½
Tomato juice, small glass			25	5½
Low-calorie minerals			0	0
Low-calorie orange squash, per oz			5	½
Low-calorie lemon squash, per oz			2	Neg

Chapter 4
Cooking and Eating for Fitness

If you want to maintain a healthy diet you must enjoy the food you eat, and to do this the food must not only taste good, it must look tempting, smell tantalizing and feel satisfying! It is the smell and the velvety feel of a warm peach that attracts us every bit as much as its taste; it is the look of the crisp salads beautifully arranged in contrasting colours that makes us want to eat them and the smell of newly baked bread that makes our mouth water.

I love eating and am an enthusiastic self-taught cook. As an avid reader of cookery books and recipes in newspapers and magazines, my idea of relaxation is planning, preparing, cooking and serving meals whether they are for the family, a few friends or a dinner party for a special occasion. All this may sound very odd when you consider the fact that I have whittled my weight down from a hefty 12 stone (77 kg) and a bit to about 8 st 4 lb (50 kg) and have to be continually weight conscious. If I relax my discipline the pounds creep back with alarming rapidity and now that I am over 40 I cannot shake them off too easily.

However, unlike the person who has stopped smoking and cannot tolerate the smell of smoke, I enjoy my food just as much now if not more. I still read all the cookery writers but the fun comes in adapting and producing dishes that are every bit as delicious and nourishing but without the potentially detrimental ingredients they contained before. Another challenge that I set myself is to use the same ideas but with far less expensive though no less nutritious ingredients. The result may not be exactly what the writer intended but what is important is that it should taste, smell, look and do you good.

Decoration and colour schemes are vital too. You can transform a quite ordinary fruit salad if you decorate it with a full-blown rose (on the table or in the salad); children can be delighted by familiar foods which are coloured red, white and blue for a Jubilee party; an 18th birthday party can become a Pickwickian feast when laid out like a pub with jugs of ale! Thought and time are your most important assets, coupled perhaps with a conviction that life is for living! It is not nearly as difficult as it may sound.

I suppose it was not surprising to find that the members of the Slimnastics groups almost without exception share my enthusiasm for cooking (after all it was over-indulgence which brought many of them to Slimnastics in the first place!). This chapter could not have been put together without their help.

The Golden Rules for Healthy Cooking

Base each meal on one of the following protein-containing foods:

> Lean meat, poultry or offal
> White or oily fish (drained of oil)
> Eggs
> Cheese (but not cream cheese – see the Food-for-fitness Calorie Tables, pages 94–102)

> Make the most of vegetables, salads and fruits in season.
> Use herbs, spices and seasonings.
> Pay attention to colour combinations and decoration.

Restrict:

Fat – butter, cream, margarine, salad oils and all cooking fats. *Never* fry.
Sugar – if you must sweeten the food use a liquid form of saccharine.
Alcohol – the occasional dash of white wine or vermouth can make all the difference but remember it is the *taste* which is left in the dish not the alcohol content so if you are only using a little – use the best!

The fit cook's kitchen

If you are going to change your way of cooking you are going to have to make sure your kitchen is properly equipped to help you.
Non-stick pans are an essential if you are going to cut down your use of fat.

A grill is important since you are never going to fry.

A blender is the one gadget which I could not do without; you can make sauces, instant food drinks, soups and pâtés and much more.

Chicken and fish bricks not only aid non-fat cookery but the aroma and taste of the food improves the more you use them.

A freezer is a time- and money-saver.

A yogurt-maker saves money (but use low-fat milk to make it with).

Kitchen foil for cooking food in its own juices.

Sharp knives and an easy sharpener.

Of course you need a non-scratch spatula for pans and do not forget a tin-opener and a cork screw!

Rolls and rolls of kitchen paper (not essential but I love it!).

Do not throw away your cookery books

The recipe books you already possess probably reflect the character of your family. Look again at those faithful old recipes and rethink them. Many cookery books give recipes containing large quantities of fat quite unnecessarily. They can usually be cut down, substituted or even cut out without substantially altering the basic tastes of the dish at all. Indeed in some cases the result can prove lighter and more appetizing without the fat.

Just to give you an example of how you can adapt your favourite dishes, here is one of my starters or lunch dishes from the *Reader's Digest* 'The Cookery Year' (which incidentally is my cookery Bible!) and is for *Spinach Ramekins*.

The original recipe runs as follows:

1 lb (½ kg) spinach
1 onion
½ level dessertspoon parsley
1 teaspoon tarragon
1 hard-boiled egg
4 sardines
2 tablespoons double cream
salt and black pepper

Garnish:
hard-boiled egg
anchovies

I made the following changes: delete the hard-boiled egg in the recipe and only use the one for decoration. Substitute 1 dessertspoon low-fat yogurt for all the cream. Make sure every bit of fat is drained off the sardines and anchovies by placing them on kitchen paper.

Method for my recipe

Cook the spinach with the tarragon, parsley, chopped onion, salt and pepper in a minute quantity of water. Drain well and put into the blender with the sardines and yogurt. Beat into a pâté. Spoon mixture into four small dishes or ramekins and chill. Garnish with chopped egg in strips of white and yellow and decorate with anchovy fillets.

In this way you are left with a delicious and pretty starter but you have considerably reduced the fat content and with it the hidden calories.

Think before you cook

Low-fat yogurt can often be substituted for cream or salad cream and adds a more piquant flavour. When milk is required use the special skimmed variety which is now readily available both in liquid and in powder form.

Pastry can add considerably to the fat and starch content of a meal which means that it is often left out of our recipes. However, as well as being tempting in itself pastry does serve a very real purpose in that it traps delicious juices and seals in the flavour and aroma of the ingredients. I was very impressed with the use of cabbage leaves advocated in the popular *Cuisine Minceur*, by Michel Guerard. I have now tried them in various ways with much success. Plunged into boiling water (blanched) until they are pliable they can line a basin – take care to overlap them – for many a steamed savoury pudding or they can line a pie dish for a quiche. Vine leaves have been used for generations to make parcels of fish or meat but cabbage and lettuce leaves can be used in the same way. Foil can be useful too – it makes serving easy and each person gets the full aroma of the dish as they open their own packet.

Many dishes would be dry and uninteresting without a sauce. The usual sauces are full of danger. However this is where the blender can really come into its own and we give you several sauces and salad dressings on the following pages which serve only to enhance the dish and not your waistline!

As we have seen, added sugar is totally unnecessary to our nutritional requirements but if you are slimming or keeping your weight under control, sweet foods must be avoided except on very special occasions. However, many fresh fruits, both home grown and imported, are always available, and there is nothing more inviting than a bowl of beautifully arranged fruits. Combined with frozen fruits you can serve many different permutations of fresh fruit salad whatever the time of year. Fruit sorbets or jellies and fools can be made from fruits canned in their own juice. Even at dinner parties these days I find that so many people are becoming conscious of the way they eat that they are quite glad to find that temptation is not even being offered to them but instead they can enjoy refreshing 'afters' with a clear conscience.

So use your cookery books, continue to read the recipes in magazines and the Sunday papers, but look at them with a clear eye, cut the quantity of fat required to the bare minimum and avoid the addition of sugar and unnecessary refined starch. In the following pages we will give you some thoughts, but these are only meant to stimulate you to further ideas of your own. Do not be afraid to experiment. We do not aim to teach you to cook but we do hope to encourage you to think about food and cooking with pleasure.

Approach cooking and eating with an open mind

Like the majority of children many of us tend to be very conservative when it comes to our food. We often closely reflect our upbringing in our likes and dislikes. Not only do we inherit our family preferences for choice of food but we also carry through life the traditional foods of our country.

I am not suggesting that we can quell all prejudice overnight, but I am saying that we must try and approach eating and cooking with a more open and adventurous mind. Luckily many countries are feeling the influence of foreign cuisines and new ideas, tastes and ingredients are more readily available.

'Sensual' Cooking

Transforming good health-giving food into dishes which are beguiling to the senses need be neither expensive nor take much expertise – just a little imagination, thought and perhaps a dash of courage! However, you will find that these extra touches not only add to your enjoyment but also to the pleasure of others. They are well worth the effort.

Eye-appeal is essential

I attended a dinner party the other day where the pale anaemic looking food was served on white plates, the table was white, so were the napkins, the lighting was harsh and made the guests look tired. I cannot even remember what we ate – the whole atmosphere was so unattractive. Contrast that with the small dinner given by some far from well-off friends; there was a lovely smell of herbs and warming bread which pervaded the house when we arrived, the lighting came from candles, the table cloth was red, the paper napkins orange, a sprig of holly had been fixed to a pin and sprayed gold for each lady, the menu had been written out with humour, making quite basic ingredients seem specially chosen for the invited guests. No wonder we all enjoyed ourselves!

Colours can be used to set the mood of an occasion; red and gold give a winter glow, yellow and green feel like spring, pink gives a summer ripeness and blue is cool, oranges and browns are autumnal. Colours set the scene; Christmas, Easter, weddings (whether they are white, silver, ruby or golden), national celebrations, all are associated with colours. Colours attract; so remember the decoration of your dishes and salads and also the colours of your plates and bowls.

We usually make an effort for special occasions or to encourage children to eat the right foods, but we often neglect to take this trouble over ourselves. If our food does not look good, we may lose interest in it altogether or just pick at bits and pieces, eating a huge number of calories without noticing them at all. It is worth making each meal an 'occasion', laying out your table or tray with as much attention as if you were a guest in your own home.

The feel of food

This is important too. One of the senses is temperature change and this needs to be satisfied. In winter we love to cup a mug of hot soup in our hands, we feel warm and comforted even before we taste it. We like stews and puddings, baked vegetable dishes and steaming drinks. In fact these hot foods make no difference to the amount of heat produced by our bodies but we feel better for them. Similarly in summer, cool salads, iced drinks, sorbets and fresh fruits make us feel refreshed and revitalized. Again the ice and the cold are not necessary to our body needs; just liquid and light nourishment would do, but our feelings would be unsatisfied.

Herbs and Spices

Our senses of taste and smell are the obvious ones to want to satisfy, but how many of us make enough use of the many herbs and spices which are available. We idolize French cookery, there is an increasing admiration for Italian and Greek cooking, the love of Chinese and Indian cooking is well known. All these methods make imaginative use of the herbs and spices.

Perhaps we should go back and try some of the flavours used before foreign spices were imported. We could use some of the aromatic English plants listed by Tusser, an East Anglian farmer of 1557, which he considered necessary for the kitchen garden:

Avens, Betony, Bleete, Bloodwort, Buglas, Burnet, Burrage, Cabbage, Clarye, Coleworts, Cresses, Endive, Fennel, Mallowes, Saffron, Lang de Befe, Leekes, Lettis, Longwort, Liverwort, Marygold, Mercury, Mintes of all sorts, Neps of all sorts, Onions, Patience, Perceley, Penerial, Primrose, Poset, Rosemary, Sage, Summer Savory, Sorrel, Spinnage, Suckery, Siethes, Tansie, Tymme, Viollettes of all sorts.

How many of us use marigolds or nasturtium to decorate our salads, or primroses or violets with our fruit and yet they are found in most hedgerows and many gardens? Do we use fennel, savory, sorrel or spinach in our salads even though they are quite delicious?

Let us consider in a little more detail some of the herbs and spices together with their uses:

Herbs

Angelica: is said to be good for digestion, colds, coughs, pleurisy and rheumatism. Use for decoration, and flavouring jellies and rhubarb.

Balm (also *Golden Lemon Balm*): the lemony taste is good in poultry stuffing, fish and stews, and for summer drinks, wine cups and salads.

Chervil: an ingredient of fines herbes, it is a sweet and spicy alternative to parsley. Very good in cheese omelettes and with most soups and stews. An excellent garnish for salads. Sprinkle on grilled fish.

Chives: the delicate onion flavour enhances omelettes, salads and dressings, tomato dishes and young vegetables such as petit pois. Add at the last moment as cooking destroys much of the flavour.

Cowslips: cowslip wine is not only delicious but was traditionally used for strengthening the nerves and relieving insomnia! Use to flavour and decorate salads and fruit jellies.

Dill: a lacy, delicately-flavoured herb, best known as a flavouring for vinegar and pickles. It is however excellent with many vegetables, salads and particularly with fish.

Fennel: superb for all fish dishes, excellent in salads with cheese and in soups. Raw it has a delightful anise or liquorice flavour. The yellow/green feathery flowers are very good for decoration.

French Tarragon (not to be confused with *Russian Tarragon* which is very bland): is one of the great culinary herbs. It is particularly good with chicken and is also a good flavouring for shellfish and eggs. Add chopped fresh tarragon to any salad.

Garden Sorrel: the acid flavour is a good contrast to fish, roast pork, veal or lamb. It is a delicious salad leaf and can be cooked as a vegetable. Mashed sorrel mixed with vinegar and a little sugar makes the traditional Green Sauce for cold meats. A recipe for Sorrel Soup is on page 131.

Garlic: has been claimed to cure many ills including the effects of smoking to leprosy and smallpox! Its culinary uses are obvious and legion, from the Aioli of Provence to scenting a salad bowl. It is also said to aid the digestion but it does give an aroma to the breath!

Lovage: has a yeasty celery flavour and is good in stews, soups, salads and their dressings.

Marjoram: this is very pungent so a little goes a long way. It can be used for stews, soups, and with pork and fish. It is also good with carrots, spinach and turnips.

Mint: the very smell of this popular herb is supposed to stimulate the appetite. There are about fourteen varieties grown in Great Britain. Spearmint is the most popular and is used for mint sauce for lamb, flavouring new peas and potatoes, cucumber salads and salad dressings. Other useful mints to grow in your garden are pineapple, eau-de-Cologne and apple. They add refreshing distinctive flavouring to fruit salads and jellies.

Oregano: closely related to marjoram. Goes especially well with tomatoes and tomato sauces. Use it also for stuffing lamb, pork or chicken and also with baked onions. It is traditionally used in Italy to flavour many different pizzas.

Parsley: a traditional ingredient to fines herbes. Use liberally as a garnish for just about everything. Used fresh and uncooked it is an excellent source of vitamin C. Steamed fish and boiled chicken are enhanced by parsley sauce.

Rosemary: used sparingly it can be delicious with lamb and other roasted meats. Try burning a branch or two on your barbecue. It adds a delicious aroma to the evening as well as the meat.

Sage: is known for its digestive qualities. Because of its strong bold flavour, fragrant though a little bitter, it must be used with great care. It is very good if used with a delicate touch with poultry, especially goose and duck, and also pork.

Sweet Basil: another of the great culinary herbs. It gives a delightful odour and mildly pungent flavour and is good with all tomato dishes and sauces, eggs, fish and salads.

Sweet Bay: a bay leaf is an essential ingredient in a bouquet garni. It is essential for marinades and court bouillon. Add a bay leaf to tomato dishes, soup or sauces. Crumpled bay leaves add much to pâté and terrines.

Sweet Cicely: this herb reduces the acidity in many fruits and it is therefore very useful for slimmers. Use with fruit salads and jellies.

Thyme: another of the ingredients of a bouquet garni. Pungent, aromatic and popular, it is used to flavour stews, soups and sauces and goes particularly well with shell fish and in dishes when wine has been used. *Lemon Thyme* adds zest and flavour to egg dishes.

Wild Roses: use for flavouring and decorating fruit salads.

Winter Savory: has a peppery flavour which is delicious with fish and bean dishes. Add it chopped to dishes of cucumber, salads and pork. Savory is said to aid the digestion.

There are no set rules for using these herbs unless you are following a recipe. However, do not destroy one flavour by using too many together, use one herb at a time and with a light touch until you have fully discovered the aroma and taste for yourself. Do not keep dried herbs for too long or their flavour will suffer. Preferably use fresh herbs – most of the above you can grow for yourselves. One of the prettiest and certainly the most 'sensuous' town garden I know is a small patch entirely devoted to herbs. On a warm evening it smells delicious!

Spices

Allspice: tastes like a blend of cinnamon, nutmeg and mace plus a strong addition of cloves! Use it with a light hand to flavour fish and egg dishes, more liberally in stews, ragouts, sauces and gravies for meat and whole for pickles and marinades.

Aniseed: strongly flavoured and highly scented, it has a light pleasant liquorice flavour when used with care. It can add flavour and excitement to fish, shellfish and gammon.

Cardamom: has as much fire as ginger to whose family it belongs. Used in curry and for pickling. It goes well with oranges and with melon.

Chilli Powder: is a delicious combination of the finely-ground pods of several kinds of hot peppers, paprika, cumin seed, dried garlic and oregano. It adds a Mexican flavour to stews, meat sauces and soups.

Cinnamon: used in moderation its fragrant odour and sweet spicy flavour is the perfect foil to fish and fish sauces. Combine with pepper, ginger, cloves and mace and rub on pork or game. Add a hint of cinnamon and cloves to mustard for ham. Sprinkle it over fresh fruit with a light fingertip.

Cloves: they have a hot spicy flavour and highly aromatic scent and must be used with care. Use for pickling, pork, ham, with onions and with fruit.

Coriander: is both sweet and sour and is a favourite ingredient in hot curries. It is delicious used with pork, cheese dishes and the pulses.

Cumin Seed: is similar to caraway seed but much stronger and is an important ingredient of curries. Use it to give a delicious Mexican or Indian flavour to lamb or chicken dishes. It is also good with the pulses.

Curry Powder: you can of course buy a ready-made commercial variety, but if you want to make your own the principal ingredients should consist of allspice, aniseed, bay leaves, cardamom, cinnamon, cloves, coriander, cumin, dill, fennel, garlic, ginger, mace, mustard, nutmeg, black pepper, white pepper, red pepper, paprika, poppy seeds, saffron, turmeric, and any others you might like! The making of real curry is passed on from generation to generation – the best help is to be taught by a friend who is already skilled.

Ginger: is a fiery spice. It is very good when rubbed on steaks and lamb chops before grilling. Use a pinch on melon and other fruits.

Mace: comes from the kernel of the fruit of the nutmeg tree. Use with fish, shellfish, eggs and some vegetables, in particular cauliflower and carrots.

Mustard: there are many different blends of mustard and many different made-up commercial brands all of varying strengths. You need to experiment to choose the brands which suit your palate. Use to flavour sauces and red meats. Use in salad dressings.

Nutmeg: can be used in the same way as mace. It is a delicate but at the same time a very aromatic spice.

Paprika: is the mild sweet cousin of the red pepper and adds colour and flavour to eggs, seafood, and vegetables. It can also be used with chicken and veal, and sprinkled on fish dishes, soups and cheese dishes.

Pepper: is for me the most essential spice in my kitchen.

Green peppers are excellent for pâtés, terrines and beef steaks.

Black pepper needs to be ground with a mill when needed for the best flavour. It adds flavour and excitement to most foods.

White pepper is less pungent and less aromatic and is perfect for light dishes.

Red pepper is very hot indeed. Use it sparingly to add excitement to fish, shellfish and salad dressings. Very good for curry and barbecue sauces, hot stews and ragouts.

Saffron: is very special and expensive. It is much used in Spain and adds the colour and zest to paella and other national dishes. Use it in fish stews and soups and rice dishes of any kind.

Turmeric: made from the dried root from a plant of the ginger family, it has a more discreet taste but it can be used to give a rich yellow colour to pickles and curries. It is added to mustard powders.

Vanilla pods: these give a subtle and delicate taste to fruit.

As with herbs, the art of combining food and spices has to be learned by the cook. It may take a little patience and courage but it will be very rewarding.

Cook to Suit Your Pocket

It is an 'old wives' tale' that living on a healthy diet is expensive. You do not need to use top quality meat and fish or vegetables that are out of season. It is the way you cook the cheaper cuts of meat that is important, the food value is just as good. You can make superb stew in the pressure cooker using inexpensive meat, stock or a tin of tomatoes as liquid and adding a variety of vegetables. There must also be at least a hundred ways of cooking mince. If there are traces of fat in the meat just make sure you cook it in advance and then you can skim off the offending fat before reheating. Cheaper fish can be baked slowly in a fish brick with orange or lemon juice plus herbs. Boiling fowls can be slowly stewed and used in cold curry sauce, salads or the flesh can be marinaded overnight in lemon juice. You can use the stock as a basis for soups and other stews.

Make the most of vegetables in season, not only for salads which we discuss later, but also when cooking. Bake potatoes in their jackets (much of the goodness is in the skin), steam onions, parsnips, and globe artichokes (in their skins too) for full flavour, cook green vegetables for the minimum time not only to avoid shrinkage but also to retain the maximum goodness. Some vegetables such as cauliflower, mushrooms, spinach can be cooked in a small quantity of skimmed milk and when just cooked, whisked in a blender and served in a purée. The whole taste is unbelievably good.

If you have a garden – of any size – use it. One of the most surprising gardens I have ever visited was in Germany. The house which was attached to a mill looked as if it had a typical neat colourful garden, but much to our amazement all the 'flowers' turned out to be edible. The border, all red and white, was Alpine strawberries, backed by rows of everlasting spinach, the bushes were red, black and green berries – all delicious, the flowers which were dotted around looked good with their backing of cabbages and carrot-tops, the trees and climbers all bore fruit. No space was wasted and in the porch were trays of seedlings waiting their turn to be planted out!

Really enjoy each fruit as it comes into season. There is nothing to beat good fruit in its prime – a glowing orange, a crisp apple, an abundance of soft fruits. Avoid the use of sugar as much as possible. Orange juice added to strawberries brings out the flavour as well as doing away with the need for added sweetness.

If you have a garden you can of course grow extra fruit and vegetables for storing in the freezer. But a freezer can be a great help even if you have no garden, live by yourself or are a small family. You can make several dishes when the ingredients are at their least expensive and store them in the freezer for further use. You can buy in bulk too, shopping at the markets or buying meat direct from the farmer or wholesale butcher. It is often fresher and the taste is better. Food is not spoiled by freezing but nor is it improved. You will get out the food you put in!

If you are on your own it is often difficult to buy small quantities of some goods and sometimes food is eaten just to avoid wastage.

This is when the freezer can come in useful. You can pop the extra into a bag and freeze it until you really need it. It can save the calories too when you are making puddings, cakes or goodies for special occasions. If you leave any leftovers lying around they beg to be eaten. Put them quickly into the freezer and remember that frozen food takes time to thaw! Another tip is to make ice cubes from real unsweetened fruit juice. Then there is always a refreshing titbit to suck when the going gets hard.

Do not turn your nose up at store-cupboard foods – with careful thought you can make nutritious and delicious meals. Tuna fish (well drained) is excellent hot or cold in salads; sardines and pilchards (again well drained of oil) add the essential calcium and vitamin D; soyabeans made up into mince or stew adds good protein and very little fat. It is important to check your cupboards so that in an emergency you will not be 'forced' to revert back to unhealthy fattening foods. For instance, tins of fruit should never be in syrup but always in their natural juices.

Another way of saving money is to live off the land. It is worth investing in one or more of the excellent paperbacks which deal exclusively in food which is to be had for free. I am continually amazed that so much goodness lies discarded, untended and overlooked around our shores, in the hedgerows and even in our gardens. There is a harvest of proteins and vitamins which are just waiting to be gleaned, fish and shellfish, seaweed and hedgeweeds, berries and nuts, herbs and salads. All you need is a well-illustrated book which tells you how to find and cook these delicacies, many of which were much prized in bygone times.

Nourishing Meals Throughout the Day

Now we have thought about the ideas in general, we hope to give you more help with the particular. We know from the members of our groups that it is often difficult to think of ideas for breakfast, lunch, packed meals, high teas and suppers, so we have given you more detailed thoughts on these. Your Slimnastics groups will give you many more; so will magazines and books. Keep reading and keep talking.

Breakfast

The first meal of the day is the most important. It is literally our 'break fast' and gives us energy and stamina. If it is your habit to snatch a quick cup of coffee and tackle the day without the aid of any sustenance, it is no wonder that you succumb to a 'mid-morning low' – this is the time that people reach for that small bar of chocolate in the mistaken belief that it will give them long-term energy. That kind of snack will give you only a temporary lift, and it will also account for approximately 300 calories! Compare that with our healthy sustaining breakfast ideas below and we hope you will be persuaded that breakfast is a *must* and it is worth getting up those few minutes earlier.

However, we do realize that life these days can be a rush and that some people cannot face cooking or even in some cases any food at all – so we have catered for them too with some uncooked breakfast ideas and some instant nourishment in the form of muesli and blender drinks.

COOKED BREAKFASTS

½ grapefruit
1 egg poached on 1 slice toasted wholewheat bread
1 small glass orange juice
tea or coffee with milk

1 slice melon
2 oz (57 g) lean bacon (grilled)
2 oz (57 g) mushrooms (grilled)
1 small slice toasted hi-bran with scraping of butter
black coffee

1 kipper grilled
1 slice wholemeal bread with scraping of butter
tea or coffee with milk

UNCOOKED BREAKFASTS

small carton plain yogurt with lemon juice
2 crispbreads with scraping of butter and yeast extract
1 oz (28 g) Edam cheese
1 small glass tomato juice

1 oz (28 g) muesli (see recipe) with ½ pint (284 ml) milk and rhubarb
stewed in orange juice
1 thin slice cooked ham
1 large glass orange juice

segments of orange and grapefruit (no sugar)
2 crispbreads with 2 oz (57 g) cottage cheese
1 glass milk

All the above contain 300 calories or less.

MUESLI

A very adequate and healthy breakfast can be contained in a bowl
of muesli. So many of the brand products are very high in their sugar
content it is preferable to buy the variety available from the health
food shops or make your own:

8 oz (227 g) rolled oats
2 oz (57 g) natural bran
2 oz (57 g) dried fruit
4 oz (113 g) wheatflakes
2 oz (57 g) wheatgerm
2 oz (57 g) unsalted nuts

Shake all these together in a container. One tablespoon weighs 1 oz
(28 g). Two tablespoons with added fresh fruit and a little milk or
low-fat yogurt (plain) will provide a good breakfast.

INSTANT BREAKFASTS

Under 200 calories:
1 whole orange (peeled)
juice of 1 lemon or grapefruit juice
1 raw egg

200 calories:
½ cup low-fat milk/yogurt
½ cup unsweetened orange juice
½ banana
1 raw egg
pinch of cinnamon

Both of these can be whisked in two minutes and will give you

stamina for hours. Do not be put off by the thought of the raw egg –
they are both delicious. You may be able to concoct others which
suit your own tastes, but remember to check the calorie content with
our Calorie Tables (see pages 94–102).

Lunch

The mid-day meal can mean many different things. It may mean a
cooked meal at home with the children, a meal on a tray by yourself,
a packed lunch at school or in the office, a snatched meal in the car
or on the run between jobs, a cheery session in the pub or a lengthy
business lunch. Without care they can all add up to too many
calories. Ideally lunch should provide about 600–700 of our day's
calories if we are keeping an eye on our weight, 300–500 if we are
actively slimming.

Just to demonstrate how deceptive snacks can be – a light snack
consisting of a sausage roll, fruit yogurt and a can of Coca-cola adds
up to 480 calories, whereas a cooked meal of grilled fish, white sauce,
carrots, green beans and a portion of fresh fruit could account for
only 280 calories. The snack was 200 calories more and it was
unsatisfying!

Meals 'on the run' when you are snatching at small amounts of
food and doing ten things at once, can be very deceptive. You will
end up convinced that you have eaten practically nothing at all when
in fact you may have consumed bits and pieces which together add up
to almost half your total calorie allowance for the day. Eating in a
hurry can cause indigestion and dyspepsia. Make every effort to
make each meal an occasion and the excuse for a short break with
time to reflect.

Recent evidence has shown that the usual 'pub' lunch, such as
sausage rolls combined with crisps and beer, can produce even more
harmful effects on the body. At about half past four following a
lunch-time visit to the pub there may be symptoms such as a sense
of undue fatigue, lack of concentration, an increasing tendency to
errors of judgement, headache, inner trembling and a feeling of
anxiety. This is due not so much to a hangover caused by the amount
of alcohol consumed but to a drop in the blood-sugar. It can be
produced by a small amount of alcohol in combination with starchy
and sweet foods. Sweetened drinks added to the alcohol, such as tonic

in the gin, result in the same effect. The obvious answer is to be sure to eat protein if you wish to drink. But do not forget that although bad effects will be reduced, the calories of the alcohol will still remain!

COOKED LUNCHES

4 oz (113 g) grilled haddock or cod with tomato sauce (see page 128)
carrots and green beans
1 small baked potato

4 oz (113 g) grilled gammon topped with a ring of pineapple
grilled tomato
2 tablespoons sweetcorn
1 baked apple (no sugar)

2 egg omelette filled with 3 tablespoons mixed vegetables
small carton plain yogurt with fresh fruit

cooked chicken quarter with mixed salad
1 teaspoon slimmers' salad dressing (see page 128)
1 banana

½ pint (284 ml) onion soup with 1 oz (28 g) grated cheese toasted on 1 slice wholemeal bread
an apple and an orange

2 frankfurter sausages with a grilled tomato
4 tablespoons peas
1 banana

All the above contain approximately 350 calories.

Lunch on your own

If you have shopped imprudently when you were tired, hungry or even perhaps feeling depressed, your larder, fridge, or store cupboard may be bulging with a tempting yet unwise selection. If you shop regularly though not too frequently at a time when you are not rushed and preferably not accompanied by hungry children, you will be able to buy carefully and selectively. This means that in those moments of 'weak will' and 'low spirit' the forbidden delicacies will simply not be close at hand to raise your spirits though only for a moment.

THE PERFECT LUNCH AT HOME – AN OPEN SANDWICH

One slice of wholemeal or granary bread, thinly spread with margarine or butter (you can also cut out the fat and moisten with tomato sauce).

1. Lettuce, hard-boiled egg, sliced, twist of cucumber.
2. Cottage cheese, sliced tomato, gherkin.
3. Marmite, lettuce, cottage cheese, slice of tomato.
4. Slice of ham and coleslaw.
5. Tuna fish, raw onion rings, 1 teaspoon slimmers' mayonnaise.
6. Chopped chicken, celery, onion, slimmers' mayonnaise.
7. Lettuce, *thin* slices hard cheese, sliced tomato.
8. Hard-boiled egg chopped and mixed with raw onion and slimmers' mayonnaise, twist of tomato.
9. Lettuce, prawns, slimmers' mayonnaise, twist of lemon.

Instead of the calorie-reduced mayonnaise you can use yogurt mixed with a little ketchup or yogurt and lemon juice. Add garlic and seasoning to taste.

Packed lunch boxes for schoolchildren

Packed lunches for children are very easy to prepare but they do need some organization. It will save you time, energy and patience if you invest in a plastic tuck box with a fitting lid and a mini-insulated flask. Have a different colour for each child. If you are at all worried about the content of the school meals or have a child with weight problems, a packed lunch is an easy as well as tactful way of watching the contents of their diet. In our experience children are very conservative and will not only be content but positively insist on having the same meal day after day! Resist every impulse to win their love through chocolate biscuits! If you have had a tiff – rather put in a little note or drawing of a happy face in the lunch box – it works wonders.

EXAMPLES OF LUNCH BOXES:

1. 1 round egg sandwiches with wholemeal bread,
   1 round marmite sandwiches with wholemeal bread,
   carrot sticks, apple, milk in flask.

2. Small plastic flask of soup,
   1 round ham and swiss cheese in brown bread,
   celery and carrot sticks,
   banana.

3. 1 round peanut-butter sandwiches,
   1 round cucumber sandwiches,
   pieces of Chinese leaf cabbage,
   1 cold sausage or frankfurter,
   1 can low-calorie drink.

N.B. Boys really do need more than girls.

Office lunches

Again organization is the key. It is probably less bulky to use plastic bags and sealing film to transport your packed lunches but a mini-thermos is a good investment and will save you pounds. To avoid gathering all the wrong foods together in a last-minute panic, you will save energy and calories if you put your lunch together the night before and keep it in the refrigerator. If you are taking an orange, ugli, mandarine or grapefruit for dessert, peel it the night before and put it in a sealed plastic bag. Remember to take a paper napkin with you!

For each sandwich use 2 thin slices of wholemeal bread from a large loaf lightly buttering one slice only, add one of the following fillings:

1 hard-boiled egg, 1 teaspoon slimmers' salad cream, watercress
3 oz (85 g) cottage cheese, 1 ring pineapple (chopped)
2 oz (57 g) shrimps in yogurt dressing, lettuce
2 oz (57 g) lean tongue, sliced cucumber
1½ oz (43 g) grated cheese with lettuce, cucumber and tomato
1 oz (28 g) cold roast beef, horseradish sauce.
plus 1 piece fresh fruit

plus in summer low-calorie soft drink or squash with ice in thermos
   in winter low-calorie or home-made soup or bouillon in thermos

All the above are approximately 320 calories which includes the bread and fruit.

You can further cut the calories in the lunches by using bread from a small loaf – this would take 40 calories away from each sandwich or by using one of the slimmers' breads – this would take away 60 calories.

If you need to cut the calories still further you can pack the ingredients in a small yogurt or cottage-cheese container and eat them with a fork.

Eating in the canteen

Canteens are usually well aware that members of their staff are health conscious – it is up to you to choose wisely. Steer clear of made-up dishes high in fat and starch, avoid the rolls and butter, choose the fruit instead of the puddings. Tell your friends that you are taking care and they will keep a close watch on you – then it is impossible to cheat! Fish or meat, salad or one vegetable, fresh fruit or plain yogurt, tea or coffee and it is as good as at home. Perhaps better as there is no temptation to 'pick'.

Eating out

It is sometimes easier to be careful over your diet when you are eating out as once you have declined something, it really does not come. You can apply the same rules as eating in the canteen.

Decline the roll!

Choose a low-calorie starter (no sauce).

Sometimes it is safest to choose another starter as a main course.

Choose a grill or poached second course – no sauces, no pastry.

Ask for a salad instead of potatoes.

Request that no chips be put on your plate (once they are there they are irresistible).

Only one glass dry white wine.

Unless it is a very special occasion – no desserts, no cheese, just coffee.

High-teas and suppers

Children back from school

They come back ravenous and often tired and bad tempered, you have to produce something appetizing and satisfying fairly quickly or they will be filling themselves up with bread and cereals! We give you plenty of ideas in Chapter 8 which will help you, so read that section too.

BAKED POTATOES

These are nearly always popular with children and can be made with various fillings. Try this one with cottage cheese and ham.

1 large potato
1 oz (28 g) cooked ham, chopped
4 oz (113 g) cottage cheese
salt and pepper
½ level teaspoon made mustard
watercress or mustard and cress to garnish

Scrub potato. Thread on to a skewer (this saves cooking time as the metal conducts heat into the centre), place it in the oven (400°F, 200°C, Mark 6) and bake until tender – about 40 minutes. Cut in half when soft to the touch, scoop out the potato and mix with the ham, cheese and seasonings. Pile back into the potato shell and re-heat for 5 minutes. Garnish with cress.

Other fillings you can try: chopped onions, 1 oz (28 g) grated hard cheese, tomato sauce with a frankfurter sausage.

LIVER KEBABS WITH BAKED BEANS

This is one of the ways to serve liver to your child without any fuss. They like to make up their own ndividual skewer.

small cubes of lambs' liver
chipolata sausages cut into small pieces
2 oz (57 g) mushrooms with small heads
small tomatoes (if liked)

Thread alternate ingredients on to the barbecue skewer and cook under the grill. Serve with baked beans.

Kebabs can also be made with kidneys, tender beef or lamb. In the summer of course they are especially enjoyable cooked outside on a barbecue grill.

On your own

Coming back to an empty flat after a hard day's work, it is quite an effort to cook a nutritious meal just for one. Also if you are retired or on your own at home all day, it often does not seem worth the effort to cater for yourself. However, eating well *is* important if you want to remain healthy and lively. If you do not feed yourself properly you are liable to put on weight – tucking into those biscuits as you watch television, do the crossword or read the latest thriller late into the night.

Either of the above recipes would suit you well but for something rather more special try one of these:

FISH BAKED IN FOIL

Any of your favourite fish responds well to this treatment. Fish is an excellent source of protein and this is one of the best ways of cooking it for slimmers, as you retain all the goodness and no extra fat is needed.

You can use trout, herring, any white fish (particularly cod, fresh haddock, turbot or plaice). Wash the fish thoroughly and place it on the foil square big enough to make a parcel. Add seasoning and a few herbs (chopped parsley, chives, dill, fennel), seal the foil parcel and bake in the oven for about 20 minutes at 350°F, 175°C, Mark 4. Chopped mushrooms and prawns or a mixture of stewed chopped onions and tomatoes can be added to the fish before parcelling it up.

For a very special occasion add 1 teaspoon lemon juice and 1 teaspoon vermouth with dill and garlic.

Serve with a salad.

COTTAGE CHEESE OMELETTE

2 eggs
1 tablespoon water
¼ teaspoon dried mixed herbs
salt and pepper
2 oz (57 g) cottage cheese
¼ level teaspoon made mustard
1 tablespoon chopped chives
small knob margarine

Beat together the eggs, water, herbs and seasonings. Mix together the cheese, mustard and chives. Melt the butter in an omelette pan (or preferably just grease a non-stick pan). Pour in the beaten eggs; stir gently, drawing the mixture from the sides to the centre in the usual way. When the egg has set, top with the cheese mixture and cook for 1 minute until golden underneath. Fold over the omelette, turn on to a warm dish and serve immediately.

You can use different fillings for this dish too. Chopped ham, tomatoes, 1 oz (28 g) grated hard cheese, prawns.

CREAMED KIDNEYS

2 lambs' kidneys
2 pints (1·1 l) beef stock
1 oz (28 g) mushrooms wiped and sliced
¼ teaspoon tomato paste
½ teaspoon made mustard
2 pints (1·1 l) low-fat plain yogurt
salt and pepper
Worcester sauce/soya sauce (dash of dry sherry on special occasions!)

Pour boiling water over the kidneys and leave to stand for 30 minutes. Skin, cut into quarters and remove the cores. Put in pan with the stock, mushrooms and tomato paste. Cook covered for 20 minutes or until just tender. Stir in the yogurt, mustard and seasonings to taste. Serve on a bed of blanched (1 minute in boiling water) bean-shoots and sprinkle with chopped parsley.

COTTAGE CHEESE SURPRISE

It may happen still, but certainly in days of old when tribes met together in the desert they traditionally feasted together in friendship. Because food was naturally scarce they pooled together all the yogurt made from the milk of their goats and into this they chopped up any other foods which were available – eggs, nuts, dried fruit, vegetables and seasonings. We can follow their example and produce an instant, healthy, nutritious but delicious supper dish for practically any number of people.

As the base use a mixture of low-fat plain yogurt and cottage cheese. Into this put (all chopped very small): hard-boiled eggs, hard cheese, apples, sultanas, dried fruit of any kind, celery, radishes, fennel, nuts, chives, onions, fresh fruit – you name it, you chop it! Season with plenty of garlic, salt and pepper.

For a change add pickled herring or smoked mackerel, again cut small.

Salads

Salads are for anytime; they can be an accompaniment to a hot dish, a starter, a satisfying main course, a combination of fruit and vege-tables; they can be plain or made aromatic with herbs, they can be conventional or exotic. A salad reflects its creator. However a salad is always a mixture of ingredients and can be made from a huge variety of vegetables and fruits both raw or cooked and combined with meat, poultry, fish, cheese, eggs or nuts. All the nutrients you need are present and in a most appetizing form – protein, vitamins in abundance, roughage and the minimum amount of carbohydrate and fat. They have the added attraction for slimmers in that raw vegetables are very filling – you can be satisfied with much less! They are economic too – expensive proteins such as shellfish can be stretched considerably by serving them in a salad.

Nearly all vegetables can be made into salads in their raw state particularly those low in calories (only potatoes and beetroot have to be cooked and these should be strictly limited by slimmers any-way!) so that you can make salads all the year round. You can be adventurous too and use wild vegetables and flowers such as dande-lion leaves, sorrel, watercress or fungi. You can appeal to the eye by decorating your salads with primroses, cowslips, nasturtium or fennel; you can contrast the colours using such vegetables as red and green peppers, or fruits such as tangerines added to chicory or strawberries with cucumbers. You can suit your own and your family's tastes. You can appeal to their sense of smell by adding delicious fresh herbs such as the different mints, parsley in quantity, chopped chives or dill.

However you make up your salads, it is the preparation of the salad that is all important. In the first place the ingredients must be fresh and in tip top condition (the tired limp lettuce leaf has put many an Englishman against such 'rabbit food'); it must be well washed and crisp. If you are using hard vegetables such as carrots, white or red cabbage, celeriac or onions they need to be shredded very fine to make for easy eating and digestion. Fruit and vegetables which quickly discolour such as apples, avocado or cauliflower need a good soaking in lemon juice.

It is the salad dressing which is the undoing of many a conscientious slimmer. A light, nutritious, appetizing salad meal can add up to a considerable number of calories if it is doused with an oily mayonnaise. If you think it is imperative to have a thick creamy sauce, serve it separately and also serve a light refreshing dressing.

SLIMMER'S SALAD DRESSINGS

1. Plain low-fat yogurt, lemon juice and herbs to taste.

2. Can of tomatoes, lemon juice, capers, garlic and herbs to taste put in a liquidizer.

3. Buttermilk and chopped mint.

4. Cucumber, yogurt, lemon juice and mint.

Recipes

It is thought and preparation together with a warm welcome which make guests feel comfortable and cherished. Entertaining should be a joy. There is no need for it to be too expensive or complicated.

It is with these thoughts in mind that we have chosen the following menus from the lunches prepared by the members of the Thursday Slimnastics group. They are varied and balanced and show especially imaginative use of herbs, spices, colour and ingredients. These are the dishes we especially enjoyed, we hope you like them too.

As we have these menus at lunch-time we do not have wine (except occasionally for a special celebration) but a chilled white wine would go well with all of them. Nor do we ever have a sweet for obvious reasons, though for a dinner party we would suggest baskets of fruits in season decorated with flowers or leaves, soft fruits of course when they are in abundance, or tins of fruit in natural juice with the addition of fresh fruit if it is scarce. We would also add home-made brown wholemeal rolls. They are easy to make, perfume the house with a delicious inviting aroma, and add a little (but healthy) bulk to the meal for those who need it.

Adrienne's menu

Adrienne loves entertaining and has a special gift for creating a warm atmosphere combined with an instinct for caring for each person individually. However, Adrienne also loves her food and this can register on the scales! We weigh in the bathroom, but even taking up one of the tiles the evenness of the floor is slightly suspect. We exercise in the spare room and half-way through are tantalized by the smell wafting up the stairs!

AVOCADO SALAD

2 avocado pears
½ grapefruit
3 oranges
5 sticks of celery
8 oz (227 g) prawns
lemon juice
french dressing
watercress

Peel and stone avocados and slice or cut into small squares. Toss in lemon juice. Peel oranges and grapefruit and slice or chop. Cut celery into ¼-in. pieces. Toss all these together with french dressing. Sprinkle with prawns and serve on bed of watercress.

PORK CHOPS WITH CABBAGE
    4 lb (1·8 kg) white cabbage, shredded
    1 pint (568 ml) low-fat natural yogurt
    8 pork chops, trimmed of all fat
    a little cooking oil
    salt and freshly ground black pepper
    sage
    4 tablespoons dry white wine (60 ml)
    2 oz (57 g) grated hard cheese

Put the shredded cabbage into boiling salted water; bring back to the boil for 3 minutes. Drain. Add the yogurt and some pepper and toss the mixture lightly. Place half the cabbage in a casserole large enough to take the chops in a single layer or use two smaller casseroles. Brush chops with oil and grill lightly on both sides. Arrange on the cabbage and season. Add a sprinkling of sage and the wine. Cover with the remaining cabbage. Cook in the oven at 350°F, 175°C, Mark 4 for about three-quarters of an hour. Just before serving, sprinkle the top with the cheese and pop under grill.

Serve with carrots, tossed green salad and baked potatoes if desired.

Angela's menu

You are quite unprepared for the imaginative living-room/dining-room/kitchen into which you step immediately on opening the front door. It is a lovely room in which to do exercises; we weigh on the kitchen floor and, although the room is small, the arrangement gives more than enough room for the nine of us. Angela has two teenage daughters, a part-time job in a hospital and does professional basket-work weaving. She is well aware of food values but even her weight creeps up in the holidays and she welcomes the constant check.

MACKEREL PÂTÉ
    1 lb (0·5 kg) smoked mackerel fillets
    2 oz (57 g) cream cheese and chives
    1 dessertspoon horseradish sauce
    1 tablespoon yogurt
    8 oz (227 g) cottage cheese
    juice of ½ lemon
    black pepper

Skin and bone fish. Put all ingredients in a blender and blend until smooth.

Serve with crispbread.

LIVER STROGANOFF

2 lb (0·9 kg) lambs' liver
4 oz (113 g) mushrooms
2 onions
2 green peppers
1 pint (568 ml) low-fat yogurt
1 tablespoon flour

Soften onion and pepper in margarine. Cut liver into thin strips and toss in seasoned flour. Brown pieces then add mushrooms. Stir in yogurt until heated through.

Serve with briefly cooked mange-tout.

Angie's menu

Angela's husband is in advertising and sometimes her house has a feeling of a stage set with props! Angie's husband is also a diabetic and so she has to be constantly aware of the nutritional food values. However, she is an artist and it is this ability which adds such flare to her cooking. She talks of 'just throwing together' the ingredients, but she achieves results which with even a lifetime of practice most of us would take quite an effort to produce! We weigh in the hall and exercise in the sitting-room alongside the bull-shaped leather couch!

SORREL SOUP

1½ lb (0·7 kg) sorrel leaves
2 cloves garlic (optional)
finely chopped onion
2 pints (1·1 l) chicken stock
2 egg yolks
salt and pepper

Simmer onion and garlic in stock until soft. Add leaves torn into pieces and liquidize all in the blender until smooth. Simmer for 10 minutes (add salt and pepper to taste). Just before serving, mix 2 tablespoons soup with 2 egg yolks in a cup then add to soup. It's important that soup is not actually boiling while or after you do this, or it will curdle.

LAMB KORMA

2 lb (0·9 kg) cubed lamb
2 medium onions
½ pint (284 ml) low-fat yogurt

6 cardamom pods (seeds)
2-inch piece of fresh ginger (if available)
a pinch of cayenne pepper
1 teaspoon salt
2 cloves garlic
1 tablespoon whole coriander seeds

} Liquidize together with ½ chopped onion and a little cold water.

Rub meat with spice purée and leave for at least 1 hour. Brown meat cubes and chopped onion in fireproof pan with a little oil if necessary. Add yogurt a little at a time so that it is all absorbed into the meat, then put covered pan in a low oven for 1 hour. Adjust seasoning.

Garnish with fresh coriander leaves if available. This was served with a fresh salad and:

CAULIFLOWER PURÉE

1 cauliflower
½ pint (284 ml) skimmed milk
grated nutmeg or ground mace
salt and pepper

Break cauliflower into pieces and add to boiling skimmed milk. Add pinch of grated nutmeg or ground mace. Cover and cook until soft. Drain and liquidize with a little of the milk to required consistency. Season to taste.

Diana's menu

We did not knock the walls down between our two living-rooms with the express purpose of running Slimnastics groups at home, but it has come in very useful! We are fortunate to have a round table as this makes for much better conversation. Our garden table is also round so in the summer we eat outside. I have two classes before the Lunch-time group so my meal has to be prepared in advance the night before or be easily assembled at the table.

MOULES MARINIÈRE

8 pints (4·5 l) mussels
5 tablespoons dry white wine
1 tablespoon each parsley, chives and dill
oatmeal
black pepper

Wash the mussels in cold water, scrub the shells thoroughly, rinse several times to remove all grit and pull or scrape away the beards. Discard any mussels with broken shells and any which remain open. Leave overnight in a bucket of cold water. Sprinkle some oatmeal on the top. The mussels will plump up and expel any undesirable waste. Rinse them once again before cooking.

Cover the bottom of a large frying pan with the wine, place all the mussels in the pan at once and cover with a lid. Place over a high heat and shake the pan for 3–5 minutes until all the mussels have opened. Take the pan from the heat, lift out the mussels into soup plates, discarding any which have not opened. Strain the liquid, add the herbs and pepper, pour over the mussels and serve immediately.

RED BEAN BEEF SALAD

2 large tins red beans (drained)
2 lb (0·9 kg) lean cooked beef, diced
2 large globes fennel
1 jar small gherkins
1 red pepper, blanched and chopped

For the dressing:
1 tin tomatoes (drained)
2 teaspoons capers
lemon juice
salt and pepper

Combine all the ingredients. Make a dressing from the tin of tomatoes (drained), capers, lemon juice, salt and pepper blended together with the liquidizer. Toss the salad in the dressing and leave in the refrigerator overnight.

Serve together with salad of shredded Chinese leaf cabbage.

Fiona's menu

Fiona leads an extremely busy life. She works as a physiotherapist at a local hospital and is also the mother of young twins. She is constantly on the go but may well need to go back to the amount of sport she enjoyed before the birth of the babies. Diet alone does not seem to be the answer in getting her weight under control, though she did find she was a victim of the 'unconscious calorie consumption', a trap easily fallen into by those with very full lives; she often feels she has 'tried everything' without success and needs the reassurance and encouragement of the rest of the group to give her the will and confidence to continue trying. We admire her pluck and good nature. Fiona also has to prepare her meal in advance.

CITRUS SALAD

4 oranges
2 grapefruit
3 tablespoons fresh mint leaves, finely chopped
few drops peppermint essence

Grate the zest from one orange. Place in a bowl with chopped mint and a few drops of peppermint essence. Remove all peel and pith from the oranges and grapefruit and discard. Then, over the bowl, carefully cut between membranes to remove fruit segments. Mix well together. Leave in the refrigerator to marinate for about 1 hour or overnight. Spoon into individual glass dishes and garnish with sprigs of mint.

CHICKEN TANDOORI

8 chicken quarters

For the marinade:
1 pint (568 ml) low-fat natural yogurt
1 teaspoon ground ginger
2 tablespoons paprika

2 cloves garlic crushed
8 peppercorns
2 tablespoons tomato purée
1 teaspoon salt

Skin the chicken. Prick well with a fork. Place all marinade ingredients in a bowl and mix well. Add the chicken and make sure it is completely covered with the marinade. Cover tightly with foil and leave for 7–8 hours or overnight.

Heat oven to 350°F, 175°C, Gas Mark 4. Place the chicken pieces on a wire rack in a roasting tin and coat with any remaining marinade. Bake for 1½ hours, basting occasionally. Remove and serve garnished with lemon wedges and parsley.

Serve with a salad of chicory and tomatoes.

Helen's menu

Helen adds a Jewish flavour to our cookery and gives us many fresh ideas. Although the Jewish methods of cooking have evolved over many centuries, to our untutored ears many of her suggestions are both novel and stimulating. Many of the recipes are nutritious but slimming. Jewish cookery makes good use of yogurt but abhors the combination of any dairy product with meat. Of course shellfish is also forbidden. I include two of her recipes which make a good vegetarian meal. Helen has only a problem with her weight when she is 'uptight' about anything and then she loses it! If Helen's weight goes down we know she is worried about something – unlike the rest of us whose tension tends to make us pick at things and we put it on! Here we weigh in the 'loo' and exercise in the spare bedroom.

SLIMMERS' EGG MAYONNAISE

1 cucumber, sliced
½ pint (284 ml) low-fat plain yogurt
8 eggs, hard-boiled
4 gherkins, chopped
3 teaspoons chopped chives
1 tablespoon chopped watercress
salt and pepper

Arrange cucumber and egg on dish. Combine remaining ingredients, season to taste and pour over eggs before serving.

VEGETABLE CASSEROLE WITH CHEESE AND YOGURT TOPPING

12 small carrots, peeled and sliced
1 aubergine, 6 oz (170 g), unpeeled but sliced
½ small cabbage, 1 lb (0·5 kg), shredded
small cauliflower, 1 lb (0·5 kg), broken into sprigs
8 oz (227 g) celery, diced
5 small tomatoes, quartered
2 onions, thinly sliced
2 cloves garlic, crushed
2 oz (57 g) butter
salt and pepper
1 large can tomatoes, blended into a purée
5 fl oz (142 ml) natural, unsweetened yogurt
2 tablespoons grated Parmesan cheese

In the order given above, put all the vegetables except the sliced onions and garlic into a large casserole dish. Cook the onion and garlic in the butter until golden. Add the tomato purée and heat through. Season and pour over the casserole. Bake for 30 minutes, or until tender but still crisp. Remove the casserole from the oven and pour yogurt over the top. Sprinkle with grated Parmesan. Return to the oven to brown slightly – or place under a hot grill for a few moments.

Jane's menu

Ever since an abdominal operation some years ago Jane's weight problem became acute. She is an excellent tennis player and the extra weight was not only unbecoming but hampering. She attended a Slimming Club and for a time lost weight steadily but found it impossible to go on with their diet. She really understands food values and weight control but it was not until she started in a demanding and interesting job that she really managed to maintain the loss. Gradually her regained looks and energy were an added incentive. She produced the following meal as a celebration!

FRESH TOMATO AND COURGETTE SOUP

2 lb (0·9 kg) skinned tomatoes
2 lb (0·9 kg) courgettes, sliced but with skins left on

1½ pints (852 ml) light stock
1 very large onion, peeled and chopped
3 cloves garlic, crushed
1 teaspoon dried basil
1 teaspoon whole coriander seeds, crushed
1½ tablespoons olive oil
salt and pepper

Heat the oil in a heavy pan; soften the onion and let it turn fairly golden. Add the courgettes and crushed coriander seeds, stir and cook for 5 minutes before adding the chopped tomatoes, garlic and basil.

Pour in the stock, add some seasoning, and simmer gently with the lid on for 15 minutes. Remove the lid and simmer for a further 10 minutes. Liquidize the soup or press it through a sieve, then reheat and taste to check the seasoning.

SALMON WITH CUCUMBER DRESSING

8 salmon steaks
½ pint (284 ml) water
juice of 1 lemon
6 peppercorns
¼ teaspoon salt

To garnish:
tomato slices
cucumber slices
lettuce
lemon slices
sprigs of parsley

For the sauce:
½ cucumber cut into ¼-inch cubes
salt and pepper
1 pint (568 ml) low-fat plain yogurt
1 tablespoon chopped fresh mint
small clove crushed garlic

Place the salmon in a shallow pan and add water, lemon juice, peppercorns and salt. Cover and slowly bring cooking liquid to simmering point. Simmer for 8–10 minutes until fish is cooked. Leave to cool in liquid. Drain, and carefully remove skin and bone.

Arrange garnish on a plate and put the salmon steaks on top.

To make the sauce, sprinkle the cucumber liberally with salt and leave for 30 minutes. Brush off excess salt, cover with a plate and drain off excess liquid. Combine cucumber with yogurt, mint, garlic and seasoning.

Chill and serve with the salmon and garnish.

Judy's menu

Judy helps her husband with his catering business. She also attends many functions and dinners in connection with this work. It is not surprising that she found her weight creeping up. It was when her clothes no longer fitted that she decided something must be done. At first she jibbed at joining an all-female lunch group – girlish gatherings not being in her line! However, we persuaded her to try one session and she has enjoyed it ever since. The very nature of our meeting hardly encourages small-talk. We are given licence to discuss both food and our bodies and the amount of knowledge that is exchanged and the help given is quite considerable. Her husband has now become a health fiend and not only eats much better but leaves home every morning for a 6 a.m. jog round the park!

TUNA AND CAULIFLOWER

    2 small cauliflowers
    2 × 7 oz (198 g) cans tuna, drained
    10 oz (284 ml) low-fat plain yogurt
    2 level tablespoons snipped chives
    2 small cloves garlic – crushed
    ½ teaspoon salt
    2 teaspoons lemon juice
    ground black pepper
    ½ teaspoon dry mustard
    2 red eating apples, cored and diced, dipped in lemon juice

Divide trimmed cauliflower into tiny sprigs. Blanch in boiling water for 2 minutes, drain and plunge into cold water. Drain again. Drain oil from tuna and flake the fish. In a bowl combine the yogurt, chives, mustard, garlic, salt, lemon juice and pepper. Fold through the cauliflower, tuna and apple.

POLPETTONE (ITALIAN MEAT ROLL)

2 lb (0·9 kg) raw minced veal, beef or pork
4 eggs
garlic
1 onion
handful of parsley
salt and pepper

Stuffing:
2 hard-boiled eggs
2 oz (57 g) cooked ham
2 oz (57 g) Gruyère or Ementhal cheese
seasoning

Mix meat, eggs, chopped garlic, onion and parsley together and season. Flatten the mixture out on a floured board. In the centre, put the stuffing of hard-boiled eggs, ham and cheese all coarsely chopped.

Roll the meat into a large sausage and put in a loaf tin. Cover with greaseproof paper or foil and bake in oven for ½ hour. Remove covering and bake for further ½ hour. Serve hot or cold.

Lesley's menu

Lesley is an ex-dancer with a fragile appearance. Her Victorian home has a tranquil air that is deceptive for it is relaxation and tension control which have been Lesley's main benefits from Slimnastics. She knows a lot about food and controls her weight well, she plays tennis and golf and also skis. However, she has had problems with sleeping and tension and loves the relaxation techniques and the fun of the group. She enjoys entertaining and experimenting with food. We weigh downstairs and exercise at the top of the house which has been converted into a children's play room.

ASPARAGUS SOUP

3 large tins asparagus bits (drained)
3 pints (1·7 l) chicken stock
1 small carton low-fat plain yogurt

Drain the tins of asparagus and put in a blender with the chicken stock. Blend until smooth. Heat through. Serve in soup dishes with one spoonful of yogurt in the centre of each dish.

COD PROVENÇAL

2 lb (0·9 kg) cod steak or fillet
seasoned flour
6 tablespoons oil
2 large onions, sliced
2 cloves garlic, crushed
4 teaspoons parsley, chopped
2 tablespoons tomato purée
12 tablespoons tarragon vinegar
12 tablespoons water
2 oz (57 g) shelled shrimps
salt and pepper

Preheat oven to 350°F, 180°C, Gas Mark 4. Cut cod into large bite-sized pieces and toss in flour. Heat the oil in a frying-pan and lightly brown the fish. Transfer to a shallow casserole dish. Fry the onion and garlic, and add to fish.

Mix the parsley, tomato purée, vinegar and water together. Pour over the fish, cover and bake for 30 minutes. Add shrimps, season to taste with salt and pepper and cook for a further 15 minutes.

Serve with tossed green salad.

Eleri's fool-proof brown bread

Eleri is an ex-group member who now lives in the country where she grows and eats her own vegetables. We are all most grateful to her for this recipe.

3 lb (1·4 kg) wholemeal flour ⎤ Rub
3 oz (85 g) butter or marg ⎬ together
3 teaspoons salt ⎦ and cover.

15 fl oz (426 ml) blood-heat water ⎤ Put in
3 teaspoons brown sugar ⎬ bowl and
1½ oz (43 g) fresh yeast or ½ oz (14 g) dried yeast ⎦ cover.

Put both bowls in airing cupboard for about 15 minutes.

Using a fork, stir the yeast mixture into flour. Add 24 fl oz (682 ml) more water. Mix again with fork then knead for 3 minutes and put in 3 × 1 lb (0·5 kg) greased loaf tins. Cover and leave in airing cupboard to rise for 20 minutes. Bake at 450°F, 230°C, for 45 minutes (Gas Mark 8). Remove from tins and cool on a wire tray.

This mixture can also divide into small rolls.

Part III
Relaxation for Fitness

The most common causes of illness in modern western
society are those of abuse, disuse and misuse of ourselves.
Apart from a sound diet, good health depends on regular
moderate muscular contraction through exercise, and also
sensible muscular relaxation as we go about our daily tasks
and confront the inevitable stresses of living.

It is the combination of exercise, sound nutrition and the
control of tension which makes Slimnastics such a complete
approach to total fitness. The following chapters look at
stress and its causes, and describe our chosen method of
dealing with it: neuromuscular relaxation, or as it is more
accurately described, tension control.

Chapter 5
What is Stress?

Not all stress is bad. We need a certain amount of stress in our lives if we are to feel fulfilled, vital and active. As one doctor has put it, 'Stress is a demand on our energy and without it we should become bored, remain emotionally immature and there would be no progress in human endeavour.'

In many ways it is as taxing to health to live lives which are understressed as to live in overstressed conditions. We can all think of many examples, such as the elderly confined to a Home cushioned from the harassment of everyday life, the women with children who are unable to pursue their careers or the man pinned down to a humdrum job for the safety of a regular income. These lives show no ups and downs, no excitements, no challenges and they often result in fatigue, depression or even illness.

The right proportion of demands upon our energy keeps us looking younger, living longer and possessing an enviable '*joie de vivre*'. We need to recognize our optimum stress level and strive to achieve this. We will then profit from stress. If, however, we have more stresses than our own particular make-up is able to withstand then we will break down. Either physically or mentally, we will cry for help. It is a question of balance.

We must also realize that our ability to withstand overstress will change from time to time as the patterns of our lives change. This means that any change in our lives, either good or bad, such as marriage, children, job, home, promotion, redundancy, illness or bereavement all take their energy toll. Too many life changes in a short space of time will inevitably cause strain and tension. Whether we get a new job, a difficult relative comes to live with us, we get married, move house or go away to college, all these events need considerable adjustment irrespective of our feelings about them whether they are pleasant or unhappy.

Overstress can lead to exhaustion and we are then more vulnerable to everyday stresses of the environment such as noise, traffic, delays, the weather and particularly it seems our friends and neighbours, and families! We all know the days when we notice any banging door, and practically anything becomes an irritation when at other times we can be unaware of any interruption at all.

Everyone has their own personal 'stress level'. What is stressful for one person is not necessarily so for another and emotional stresses cannot easily be compared between one person and another, nor can they be compared in the same person in succeeding years. We need regularly to take stock and assess our own balance sheet.

How to Recognize Overstress

We have seen how overstress can lead to exhaustion. Let us look at the medical description of the changes in behaviour this condition can lead to.

Exhaustion is a fascinating and common aspect of life but it is rarely recognized and treated. Its essence is evidenced by the fact that any increase in the demands upon an individual, or any striving harder on his part actually worsens his performance. The worsening performance leads to anxiety and irritability, which in turn affect the person's performance even more. The same factors also affect sleep which aggravates the exhaustion and sets up another vicious circle of deteriorating performance. The ability to discriminate between essential and petty matters is lost when someone is exhausted – longer hours are worked but less is achieved. The exhausted individual soon becomes unfit, but he stoutly denies the personal and social disintegration that is becoming obvious to others. Commonly he eats, drinks, smokes and talks too much. A desire for stimulation may make him neglect reasonable advice to rest and 'recharge his batteries' and spurts of effort are put into 'rash bashes' of physical activity in the mistaken belief that spasmodic exercise can cure the disorder of exhaustion.*

Compare this with the description below of a man in good health and you will see the difference:

The individual feels well. His manner is relaxed and physical recreation brings pleasure and does not cause guilty reactions. Burdens and pressures that would cause loss of happiness and health are rejected. Increasing

*P. D. F. Nixon, the *Practitioner*, 1976, issue 217 (Heart), pp. 765 and 935.

stimulation enhances the performance. Other people look upon him and his relationships as healthy and see him as adaptable and approachable. The qualities required for success, namely rapid and flexible thought, originality, vigour, expansion and capacity for sustained effort are abundant.*

Most of us are somewhere between the two! But many of us can recognize the times when we have, through sheer exhaustion, pushed ourselves too far, resulting perhaps in an irrational family quarrel or a strained back brought on by insistent gardening until sundown. Unfortunately the truly exhausted are beyond taking advice either from themselves or from their friends. It is not until they are forced to visit their doctor, suffering from an illness aggravated by tension, or an infection caught through lowered resistance, or even an accident because their minds are preoccupied, that the vicious circle is broken. We need to stop ourselves before this point is reached.

Learn your 'stress signals'

We all have our own individual signs of increasing tension. We should watch out for these warning signals and learn to take avoiding action. We all have our most vulnerable spots – perhaps yours is one of these:

Throbbing head, headache or migraine,
Tightness in the throat,
Eyestrain,
Tight scalp or skin rash,
Pain in the neck or between the shoulders,
Breathing problems, even asthma,
Pains in the chest,
Twitching thumbs, fiddling fingers, clenched hands, bitten nails, damaged cuticles,
Skin problems,
Aches and pains in the back,
Butterflies in the tummy, indigestion, bowel trouble, frequent visits to the toilet.

If you have a recurring problem like this and there is no medical cause, it may well be a signal that tension is getting the upper hand.

*P. D. F. Nixon, the *Practitioner*, 1976, issue 217 (Heart), pp. 765 and 935.

Sheer willpower will not help us to overcome exhaustion; we need to counterbalance our periods of effort with relaxation. There are several ways in which we can help ourselves.

The Nervous System

Without the nervous system we would be like puppets without strings or carefully constructed robots without power. We need to learn to treat our delicate and intricate 'electrical' system with respect, as misuse can lead to 'power' failure resulting in physical or mental collapse.

In Man the nervous system is composed of the sense organs, the brain and spinal cord, the peripheral nerves and the autonomic system.

The sense organs

The skin, nose, tongue, eye and ear enable us to experience the eight sensations of pressure or touch, temperature, pain, smell, taste, hearing, balance and sight. These all detect the minutest change in our environment. Nerve impulses then carry this information to various parts of the body and we are able to react in a sensible co-ordinated way.

The brain and spinal cord

The brain is the centre of the nervous system, receiving messages via the spinal cord, correlating them, storing impressions for future use or sending our conscious or unconscious instructions, controlling our sense organs, glands and muscles. Intellectual activity takes place and thoughts and memories are carefully filed and indexed or else erased or forgotten if not of use. All this without conscious effort!

The peripheral nerves

These are the nerves over which we have direct control such as those from the brain to the arms and fingers.

The autonomic system

This system serves involuntary muscles and glands and controls two major types of behaviour, energy consuming on the one hand and rest and pleasure on the other. These two automatic counterbalancing parts are:

(a) *The sympathetic nervous system*: This branch is responsible for all those activities where you burn up energy in the muscles. They are particularly brought into play during 'fight or flight' situations such as are experienced in stress moments. Normally this system is only active as long as the muscles are working. But if muscular tension is sustained it can remain active after the need to burn energy has disappeared, leaving the tension sufferer unable to unwind.

(b) *The parasympathetic nervous system*: Your body is governed by the parasympathetic nervous system when you are eating and digesting, going to sleep, becoming sexually aroused or just relaxing. For instance in the process of digesting a meal, acid is produced by the stomach, the amount being determined by the autonomic nerves which go from the brain to the stomach, and although we are unaware of their activity, they automatically ensure that the right amount of acid is produced during and after the meal. However, the parasympathetic nervous system cannot function properly if you are tense.

Most organs of the body are affected by nerves from both the sympathetic and parasympathetic systems. The heart is speeded up by sympathetic nervous stimulation and slowed down by parasympathetic stimulation. During the early phase of sexual arousal parasympathetic activity predominates, while during orgasm the sympathetic nerves are mainly involved. These two systems act together like a sea-saw – while one is up the other must be down. This explains the reason why the activities of the parasympathetic nervous system are unable to take place properly while you are in a sympathetic nervous state.

The chemical messengers

The brain also controls the release of chemical messengers, the hormones, which regulate the glands of the body such as the thyroid, adrenals, ovaries and testes. The word 'hormone' is derived from a

Greek word meaning 'to excite' which gives a good idea of the role they play in the body in that they stimulate growth and development and activate certain types of tissue.

The many and varied glands in the human body can be divided into two categories:

(a) Those which deliver their products directly into the digestive or alimentary canal or which like sweat and sebaceous glands open on the surface of the body.

(b) The so-called ductless glands which pass their products directly into the bloodstream. The four most important of these glands or endocrine organs are the thyroid and parathyroid, the pituitary, adrenal and the gonads or sex glands. Together these glands control the metabolism of the body and any over or under activity can affect our growth, weight, appetites and behaviour. Most of the endocrine glands have an automatic feedback system, whereby if too much hormone is produced, the brain reduces the amount of the stimulation to that gland. However, as this secretion of hormones has such a profound effect on the brain, over-activity can produce irritability, depression, tension and aggression. These effects can be substantially controlled by hormone replacement under medical supervision.

It is the response of the adrenal glands to a stress alert from the pituitary gland, which is seated at the base of the brain, which is of most interest to us here. When the body is faced by an emergency or challenge the pituitary gland sends a message to the adrenal gland and extra amounts of adrenalin are released from the adrenals which are situated just above the kidneys. Within seconds of an emotional reaction adrenalin is poured into the bloodstream to prepare the body for 'fight or flight'. It makes the heart beat faster, diverts blood to limbs and brain, relaxes bronchial tubes to allow more air into the lungs; less blood flows to the digestive organs (causing those butterflies) and to the skin so we may also turn pale with fright or anger. At the same time the adrenalin transforms glycogen in the liver into glucose to provide quick energy. Fat is also released into the bloodstream so that there is another ready supply of energy available. With this power thrust into the body by the adrenalin we are able to perform physical feats we would be quite unable to do under normal circumstances.

Cortisol is also released by the adrenal gland in response to stress and it has an influence on the fluid and salt content of the body. Although this hormone, cortisone, is a defence against allergic reaction and inflammatory conditions after injury, too much can result in stomach ulcers.

The body and the brain cannot be functionally separated. They are constantly having a reciprocal effect on one another, Uncontrolled physical reaction to stress situations can result in illness or even death. To drive this point home let us look more closely at the results of this 'stress alert' in our bodies and the damage we can do to ourselves.

'Fight or Flight'

Imagine you are about to be run over by an oncoming bus – your muscles would tense (you might freeze to the spot), your heart would pound, your breath come faster, you might start to tremble and sweat, have clammy palms and butterflies in the stomach. You would be mentally very alert but literally wide-eyed with fear, your pupils dilated, and if severely frightened your bladder and bowel might empty. All this is an instinctive reaction to a real situation which needs instant energy. Tense muscles have resulted in a stress alert in the brain and the whole body has been got ready for action. These physical preparations are absolutely necessary when we are called upon to deal with some sudden dramatic situation or preparing for a challenge like running a race. However, if we prolong these reactions or invoke them unnecessarily or too frequently we can damage ourselves. We may have so many stress situations in our lives that the sympathetic nervous system stays constantly active and the parasympathetic nervous system is unable to function properly. We may also trigger off the 'stress alert' in the brain by the physical tension of our muscles giving the brain a false or exaggerated picture of our position. We may fail to notice the tightening of our fingers round the steering wheel in a traffic jam, the frowning concentration over a difficult piece of work, the clenched teeth when faced by a wilful child, the hand clutched over the arm of a chair during an exciting T.V. match – none of these may register until it results in a painful neck, ache between the shoulders, a splitting head or perhaps an upset tummy.

If the body has been prepared for 'fight or flight' it is absolutely necessary to drain off the tension by physical activity. Unfortunately civilized human beings rarely put this energy to good use. Unlike wild animals or our primitive ancestors most of us do not take physical action in times of stress. This means that the increased blood-sugars and fats poured into the bloodstream as a result of the hormone action, can simply remain there. These, it is thought, cause a build-up of deposits in the blood vessels so that coronary thrombosis is more likely to occur.

Problems Caused by Tension

Vomiting, fainting attacks, eyestrain and twitching, even temporary blindness, skin irritations or red blotches, cold sores, mouth ulcers, baldness can all be triggered off by strain caused by tension.

Angina: Anxiety and tension, unlike exercise, make the arteries of the heart constrict. Angina is pain produced by a heart muscle which is required to work with insufficient oxygen.

Asthma: Anxiety can make the small involuntary muscles of the bronchial tubes in the lungs go into spasm and produce wheezing, hyper-ventilation or even asthma in some people. (Asthma can also be caused by allergies, see page 226.)

Digestion problems such as gastric, duodenal or peptic ulcers; colitis when the bowels go into spasm and a spastic colon produces abdominal pain and constipation. Sometimes nervousness can cause diarrhoea. Anxiety can also make people want to pass urine more frequently than usual, while a severe fright may make them incontinent. Embarrassment can temporarily prevent some people being able to pass urine at all.

Fatigue and cramp: Excess acid build-up leads to tiredness and aching muscles and this can result in severe neck or back pain.

Heart attacks: Several causative factors have been clearly identified among which high blood pressure, obesity, cigarette smoking and excess fat in the bloodstream can all be aggravated by tension (see page 223).

Obesity: Memories of being comforted in childhood by being given something 'nice' (sweet) to eat can turn a tense adult to these child-hood treats. Uncontrolled this can lead to obesity.

Performance problems: Muscle tension can result in incoordination which can seriously affect those whose jobs depend on having a steady hand such as surgeons, dentists, musicians. Tension can diminish their ability to do their job skilfully and accurately. Stage fright can affect the voice because the muscles which control the vocal cords become too tight.

Resorts of the overstressed: Smoking, alcohol, drugs and tranquil-lizers can all produce illness or dependence.

Sexual problems: Anxiety can have a very bad effect on sexual functions. Incoordination of the autonomic nervous system can produce an inability to get an erection or premature ejaculation in men. Vaginismus is a painful spasm produced by anxiety in women. An inability to reach a climax may occur in both sexes. Fear of failure very soon leads to a vicious circle and loss of libido or sexual drive. Tension can also result in lack of menstruation, infertility or even spontaneous lactation.

Tension headaches and migraine can be brought on by stress. The blood pressure can rise and the arteries which supply the brain can go into spasm. Where the spasm is followed by dilation so that the nerve endings in the artery walls are stretched causing pain, this causes a pulsating headache, which in the case of migraine, usually only affects one side of the head. (Migraine can also be caused by food allergy and low blood-sugar, see page 226.)

Chapter 6
Introducing the Slimnastics Relaxation Programme

The technique we use in Slimnastics is based on neuromuscular relaxation. One of its main advantages is that it is a straightforward, uncomplicated approach to the relief of tension. Not only is it easy to understand and learn, it is simple to put into operation even under stress conditions and – most important of all – it works! At first this form of relaxation requires concentration and practice, but once it has been mastered stress symptoms will recede and it will free your physical and mental energies to deal with life and its problems as they come along. The stresses and strains will gradually come into perspective and you will be better able to deal with problems.

The purpose of neuromuscular relaxation is to switch the body into the parasympathetic nervous state. As we have seen messages are transmitted in two directions: worries, anxieties, and stresses in the brain cause tension in the muscles; tension in the muscles brings about a 'stress alert' in the brain. This means that we only have to think about a frightening or challenging situation to cause the bodily effects of a 'stress alert' to be put into operation or alternatively only maintain muscular tension to have a similar effect but this time with no conscious cause. In both cases the whole body is affected. It is with messages from the muscles to the brain that we stand our best chance of changing the situation. To put neuromuscular relaxation into practice it is essential to learn to recognize when the muscles are under tension and then to become fully aware when this tension is released.

Exercises which will help you to recognize tension

Try the following exercises, really concentrate on feeling the tension in your muscles and then the release, allowing the muscles to relax until they feel very heavy and almost detached from the body.

(*a*) Make a fist with each hand. Hold hard. Look at the white of your knuckles, feel the tension up the arms, in the shoulders, in the chest. Release. Feel heavy. Repeat.

(*b*) Lie flat on your back. Closing the eyes helps concentration. Starting at the toes and working up the body clench the muscles of the feet, calves, knees, buttocks, hands, shoulders, face. Hold, recognize the tension. Release, feel heavy. Repeat.

Tension control

Find a period in the day when you can practise your relaxation for about 15 minutes. You should consider it as important as eating, washing or cleaning your teeth! Banish any guilty feelings about inactivity, these 15 minutes are a very positive part of your healthy programme for living. Make sure your friends, family and children respect this use of your time, after all they will feel the benefits!

It does not matter what time of day you choose. You may have to vary it to fit in with your timetable. You may be able to take 15 minutes for yourself during the day, or perhaps just after you return from work. Just as long as you can be comfortable, warm and undisturbed the time and place are immaterial. For a few moments enjoy this retreat.

Practise the following neuromuscular relaxation programme lying flat with your eyes closed. You will need to memorize each section before you start. When you release the muscles after tension, allow yourself to feel the relaxation for several seconds.

The Neuromuscular Relaxation Programme

1. You are going to work slowly down the body, feeling the tension, release and relaxation in the muscles.

(*a*) *First concentrate on the muscles of the head.*

Frown hard and tense the muscles of the scalp. Hold and release.
Frown just between the eye brows. Hold, release, let go.
Screw your eyes up tight. Hold and release.
Keeping your eyes closed, screw them up as if there was a bright light. Hold and release. Let go.

Pull the mouth out slightly. Hold and let go.

Pull the corners of the mouth out taut. Hold and release.

Clench your teeth together tightly. Hold hard, release and let your tongue and your jaw drop down. Repeat.

(b) *Concentrate on your hands.*

Put your arms by your sides.

Push your palms down into the ground. Hold and release.

Clench each hand into a fist. Hold and release.

Turn the backs of the hands to the floor. Your hands are very heavy, you want to raise them from the floor but it is impossible. Try to do so and then let go.

(c) *Concentrate on your back.*

Push the small of your back hard into the ground and then release.

Arch your back and push your tummy up. Hold and then let go.

(d) *Concentrate on your feet.*

Push both heels hard into the ground. Hold and release.

Push both knees down into the ground. Hold and release.

(e) *Concentrate on breathing.*

Bend your elbows, rest your hands lightly on your diaphragm. Breathe in deeply and expand.

Exhale through your mouth, forcing the air through clenched teeth and pursed lips until the diaphragm contracts.

Continue to concentrate on your breathing, feeling yourself expand and listening to yourself exhale.

Continue to practise this every day for 15 minutes.

2. The next stage in the programme is to put this relaxation technique into practice. To start with, select a short period such as a bus ride, a family meal or an evening watching television, in which to check the tension in your muscles. When you recognize a muscle under tension deliberately tense it up still further and then release. Try to keep this muscle contraction as invisible to

others as possible, gradually the action will become involuntary and almost automatic. Nevertheless, keep checking every now and again, clear that brow, unclench that jaw, release those fists. Not only will you feel better, you will look better too!

3. The final aim is to put neuromuscular relaxation into practice in stress situations. The calm relaxed person has a head-start in any battle of wits and also possesses the ability to see things in perspective. If you can learn to relax your muscles under these circumstances your brain will 'know' there is no emergency and you will be in command of any situation.

Always make the best use of time. Lack of time is one of our greatest stressors but use time correctly and it is on your side.

(a) Arrive on time for appointments – this aids relaxation and confidence.

(b) Estimate time with allowance for handicaps (the bus that is late, the weather that delays). This will avoid panic and stress.

(c) Take your time when doing anything which normally makes you tense. Do everything slowly and carefully and then you will not be rushed into making mistakes or being anxious.

(d) Concentrate on breathing regularly and deeply, taking every conceivable measure not to hurry.

(e) Quietly check the tension in your muscles, contracting the muscles firmly and then releasing the tension into relaxation.

(f) Check your posture, sit or stand balanced but at ease.

(g) If at any time you feel the tension rising in your body check your muscles again, contract and release.

You will be ready for anything!

With muscular tension under control you will release more energy to meet the real emergencies and challenges as they come along. The added benefit of these relaxation exercises is that you will find they create a marked improvement in muscle tone and ultimately a feeling of physical as well as mental well-being and confidence.

Positive Ways to Blow Off Steam

In order to give and gain the best in our lives we need a combination of passive and active relaxation. However well you master and practise our relaxation programme there comes a time when positive physical action becomes a necessity to drain off nervous tension. We literally need to burn up the excess sugar and fats in our bloodstream and use this extra energy in movement. Bottled-up energy can lead to frustration and even violence.

Walking

Walk whenever you can. We were a much fitter race when we had to walk to school, or work, to visit our friends and neighbours. Sometimes we hardly use our legs at all, we use cars, buses, lifts and escalators. We sit at desks, over the table and lounge in front of the television. If it has been a bad day in the office, don't stand miserably at the bus stop, walk on to the next, and the next. The fresh air as well as the movement will do you good. If you have been shut in all day at home get out when you can and walk round the block or to the fields or park. You will feel much better when you come back again.

Jogging

This has been hailed as the newest rediscovery, the recommended cure-all from doctors and psychiatrists alike! There are even some doctors who believe that since we are descended from people who had to run to stay alive we have a 'genetically-programmed' need to run to stay healthy. They argue that when we neglect this activity we can suffer from depression, anxiety, constipation, headache and stomach trouble.

Well-documented clinical research for both sexes shows that exercise and jogging are an excellent way to retrain the middle-aged heart, and enable the lungs to extract more oxygen from the air we breathe. It also opens up unused 'spare capacity arteries' in the heart. This results in most people feeling revitalized. Joggers not only look better but feel good, have more stamina, less anxiety and do better in exams!

In view of the damage caused to our bodies by prolonged muscle tension and build up of adrenalin it is easy to see how beneficial jogging could be. There is, however, one word of warning – jogging should not be attempted by those who are overweight, have poor posture or who are ill-equipped! If you are heavy or have drooped shoulders, round back, large abdomen, tight chest muscles, your heart will be unable to perform well and produce the extra oxygen required by the hard working legs. This could result in strain of the heart muscle. The legs too can suffer if the posture is incorrect. Knock knees, weak ankles, can lead to torn ligaments or even varicose veins. Running in street shoes or on pavements may damage your tendons. Even tennis shoes give little support. Nor should jogging be attempted by anyone with a medical problem or condition. It is wise to check with your doctor first.

Having said all this, if jogging is for you, almost everyone who jogs feels exhilarated, works up a perspiration and feels good. Jogging does not take up much time, you do not have to join a club or have special premises, nor do you need special skills or expensive clothes. All you need is determination and a reasonably healthy body. You can wear comfortable clothes in which you can move and sweat such as a track suit or shorts and T-shirt and you will need track or running shoes which are designed to take the impact.

If you are a healthy but out-of-condition man or woman, here is a graded programme of how to get started:

First week: Jog and walk for half a mile, alternating 100 paces running with 100 paces walking.

Second week: Jog and walk 1½ miles, alternating 100 paces running with 100 paces walking.

Third week: Jog one mile at any speed that is fairly comfortable to you.

Remember to build up gradually again if you have a break, especially after any illness.

Never drink alcohol just before or after running. It stimulates the heart too much, and do not eat for 3 hours before a run or you may get indigestion.

Do stop if you have any signs of over-exertion such as pain in the chest, severe breathlessness, dizziness, nausea, or loss of muscle control. Check your pulse 5 minutes after finishing a run. If it is over 120 per minute you have done too much, so cut it down the next time.

Do not give up – the best results come from perseverance!

Swimming

This is one of the best forms of exercise for almost everyone. With the water supporting the body, swimming puts no extra strain on limbs or joints so that age, excess weight, muscle or joint problems are no bar to this form of exercise. Swimming strengthens the whole body, improves co-ordination, breathing and stamina.

Moving to music

Dancing is not only for the very young. A Chelsea Pensioner we met the other day proudly put down his obviously healthy state of body and mind to his twice-weekly visits to a ballroom dancing club!

Rhythm has a very definite effect on our state of mind. Watch the people shopping in the supermarket only vaguely aware of the music and its influence – dreamy, melodious tunes and they will be soothed into slow deliberation and extra purchases, on the other hand speed the music up and they will be marching through the tills in quick succession. Rhythm can be a dangerous thing too. Look at the tribes built up to warring frenzy by the beating drums. On the other hand we can use it to our advantage. Dance to a quick beat and your aggression will be released, sway gracefully to the classics and your soul will feel at peace.

If you are caught in at home or the weather prevents you from going out, we suggest that you have a disc or tape always at hand, ready to use when you need to 'blow your top' or raise your spirits. We have worked out a series of dances for you to use (see Fig. 15). Shut the door, close the curtains and let yourself go! Music is a marvellous healer.

Exercises

Of course all the action we have suggested above concerns exercise, but we know from members of our groups that there are times that positive exercise is needed when overt action is impossible. They are thinking of such times as office meetings (see Fig. 16), family quarrels (see Fig. 17), waiting in a traffic jam (see Fig. 18), strap-hanging in the tube (see Fig. 19), or when confined to bed (see Fig. 20). The

High Kicks for Low Spirits

Fig. 15 With or without jumping, as you wish. Dance away to your favourite music. Get the blood flowing and the body glowing.

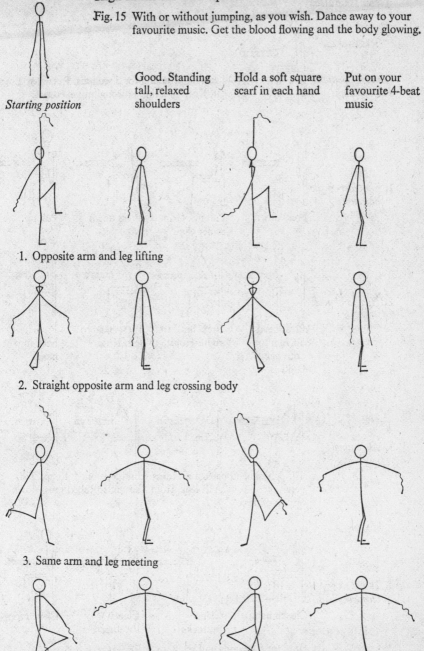

Starting position

Good. Standing tall, relaxed shoulders

Hold a soft square scarf in each hand

Put on your favourite 4-beat music

1. Opposite arm and leg lifting

2. Straight opposite arm and leg crossing body

3. Same arm and leg meeting

4. Opposite arm and leg meeting

Desk Exercises

Fig. 16

Starting position
Back straight

Hold each contraction for 5 seconds. Relax for 2 seconds.
Repeat. Keep breathing throughout exercises.

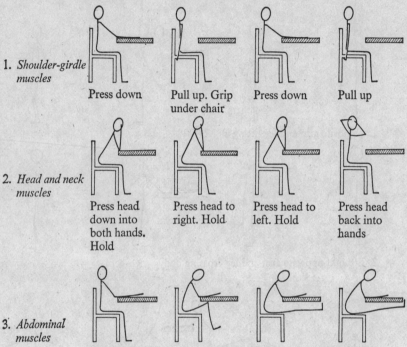

1. *Shoulder-girdle muscles*

Press down — Pull up. Grip under chair — Press down — Pull up

2. *Head and neck muscles*

Press head down into both hands. Hold — Press head to right. Hold — Press head to left. Hold — Press head back into hands

3. *Abdominal muscles*

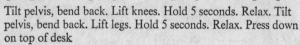

Tilt pelvis, bend back. Lift knees. Hold 5 seconds. Relax. Tilt pelvis, bend back. Lift legs. Hold 5 seconds. Relax. Press down on top of desk

4. *Hands, toes, buttocks, legs*

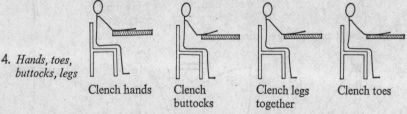

Clench hands — Clench buttocks — Clench legs together — Clench toes

Hold for 5 seconds and relax for 2. Repeat

Sequence at the Kitchen Sink

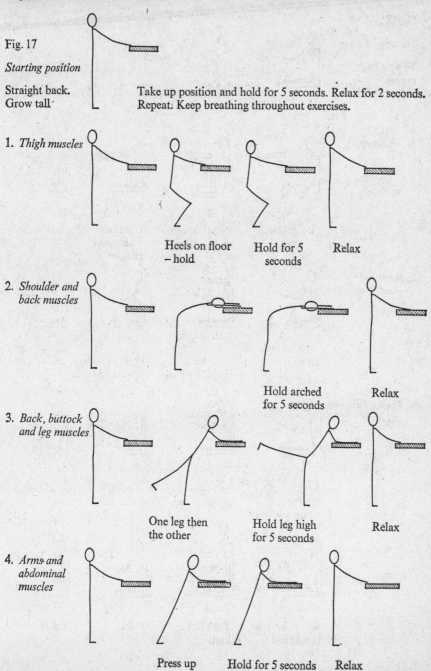

Fig. 17

Starting position

Straight back.
Grow tall·

Take up position and hold for 5 seconds. Relax for 2 seconds.
Repeat. Keep breathing throughout exercises.

1. *Thigh muscles*

Heels on floor
– hold

Hold for 5
seconds

Relax

2. *Shoulder and back muscles*

Hold arched
for 5 seconds

Relax

3. *Back, buttock and leg muscles*

One leg then
the other

Hold leg high
for 5 seconds

Relax

4. *Arms and abdominal muscles*

Press up

Hold for 5 seconds

Relax

Car Exercises

Fig. 18

Starting position

Sit well back
in seat.
Straight back

Keep breathing naturally and regularly.

1. *Abdomen*

Sit up straight   Press back into seat hard   Contract abdominal muscles   Relax

2. *Back and shoulders*

Sit up   Arch back – shoulders back   Press shoulders down and back   Relax

3. *Thighs, buttocks and arms*

Sit up, press inwards to steering wheel   Grip legs together hard   Harden buttocks   Relax. Let go

4. *Feet and shins*

Sit up, breathe slowly and deeply   Turn feet up hard   Hold   Relax

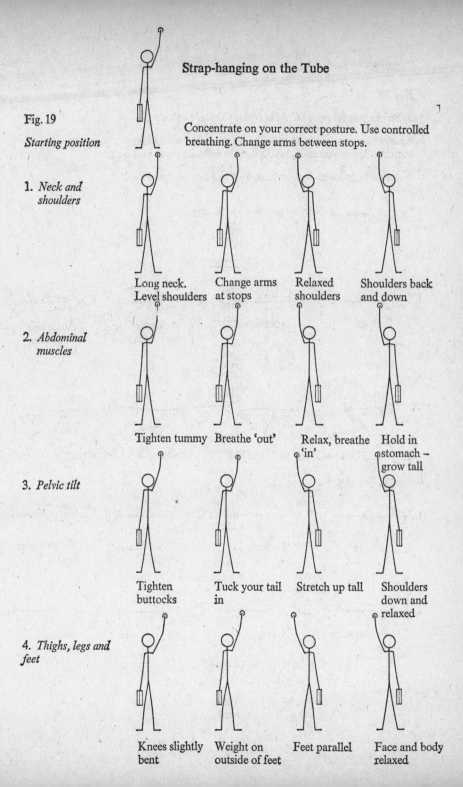

Strap-hanging on the Tube

Fig. 19

Starting position

Concentrate on your correct posture. Use controlled breathing. Change arms between stops.

1. *Neck and shoulders*

Long neck. Level shoulders

Change arms at stops

Relaxed shoulders

Shoulders back and down

2. *Abdominal muscles*

Tighten tummy

Breathe 'out'

Relax, breathe 'in'

Hold in stomach – grow tall

3. *Pelvic tilt*

Tighten buttocks

Tuck your tail in

Stretch up tall

Shoulders down and relaxed

4. *Thighs, legs and feet*

Knees slightly bent

Weight on outside of feet

Feet parallel

Face and body relaxed

Exercises in Bed

Fig. 20

a) Before you get up. *b*) Cold in bed. *c*) Tense, can't sleep.

To increase circulation, to mobilize joints and to strengthen muscles. Before you start, take 3 deep breaths slowly in and out.

Never lie in bed with legs crossed, as it stops or hinders blood flow.

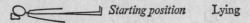 *Starting position*   Lying

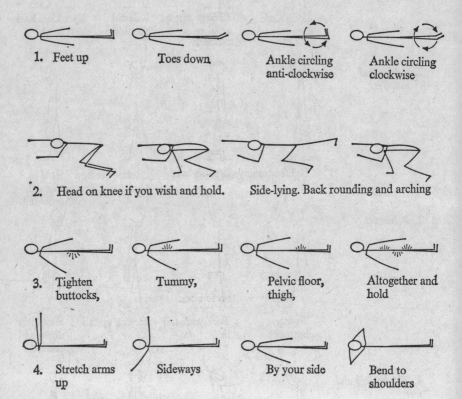

1. Feet up   Toes down   Ankle circling anti-clockwise   Ankle circling clockwise

2. Head on knee if you wish and hold.   Side-lying. Back rounding and arching

3. Tighten buttocks,   Tummy,   Pelvic floor, thigh,   Altogether and hold

4. Stretch arms up   Sideways   By your side   Bend to shoulders

Loo Exercises

Fig. 21

Squatting with thighs together and pressed against abdominal wall, supports abdominal organs and possible rupture areas during defecation. This encourages greater efficiency and less strain, less constipation (full or partial). Exercises strengthen abdominal and trunk muscles.

Starting position

Squatting, knees together, thighs touching abdomen, feet raised on stool if possible. (A low lavatory has same effect.)

IF NO STOOL, lean forward and grasp below knees, feet up on tiptoe

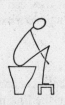

1.   Arch and round back

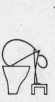 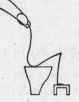 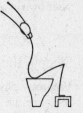

2.   With legs apart, arch and round back through legs

3.   Turn shoulders to alternate sides

   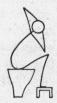

4.   Bend to alternate sides

exercises we have developed can be very useful at such times. Working the muscles strongly in opposition to one another can displace energy imperceptibly and improve the shape of the body at the same time. We have worked out a series of exercises for you to memorize and use when needed. We have also included a set of exercises to be done in the 'loo' (see Fig. 21). This seems, quite understandably, the place where many people flee in times of stress. Here they can be alone with their emotions but they can hardly let rip! So next time don't just sit there, do something – our exercises!

Sport

Naturally competitive sport both encourages and dispels adrenalin. We have mentioned several in the first part of this book. However, we have concentrated in this chapter on action that can be taken on your own at a time and place to suit yourself.

Sleep – the Most Complete Form of Rest

Vigorous physical exercise and its natural counterparts, sleep and rest, are the main factors which affect the efficiency of the heart, lungs and general circulation. All tissues, organs and bodily systems need periods of rest to alternate with periods of activity. The heart and lungs are no exceptions to this rule, although naturally they can never rest completely.

In sleep, movements are only occasional and the muscles lose most of their tone, breathing becomes slower and deeper, the pulse slows and the blood pressure falls. The sleeping body, especially when warm, needs much less oxygen than when awake and this reduces the work of the heart and lungs to a minimum. Regular hours of sleep are essential for your health and well-being but the amount of sleep required varies from individual to individual. Some can manage with as little as five hours while others need eight hours or even more. As we get older we tend to need less sleep. It is important to realize that this is an entirely natural change. Worry over lack of sleep is self-defeating!

It is the quality not the quantity of sleep that should cause concern. If we wake still tired, tense and unrested, burdened by the pressure of the day ahead we may well be overstressed and heading for exhaustion point. The sympathetic nervous system has remained active and the muscles have been unable to gather energy and restore the body to a state of calm. Insomnia or at least inadequate sleep caused by over-stress increases exhaustion and creates a vicious circle. This con-dition, if it persists, requires medical help to restore a natural rhythm and reduce fatigue.

True insomnia is unusual and indeed if you have followed the advice in this book, are eating well but moderately, taking plenty of physical exercise, working at optimum stress level (not below or above), and allowing yourself periods of rest, you are more than likely sleeping like a top. On the other hand occasional sleeplessness is something from which most people suffer. This can become a severe stress especially if you take it too seriously.

Going to bed

If sleep is a problem, the winding-down routine before you go to bed can be very important. In the first place, think about the time you go to bed. Most of us can be divided into 'larks' or 'owls', the 'larks' rise early in the morning eager to be up and getting on, the 'owls' rise sluggishly but come to life in the evening. A lark who goes to bed too late may well be overtired. The owl may be bad-tempered in the morning but he will be raring to go just as the lark turns in. Unfortunately most of our lives force us into the 'average' mould, first at school and then at work and so on through life. Somehow we have to adjust. A short 'cat-nap' can boost the flagging energy of the lark and a good physical work-out can tame the owl. We need to establish a routine to suit ourselves and those around us.

It is difficult to sleep well if you are cold. A comfortable, firm bed and a continental quilt can be the ideal combination for instant warmth and a feeling of security. Night starvation does not help either. There is some evidence to show that milky drinks really do work, but if this adds too many calories or fat to your daily allowance, try an orange (the vitamin C will calm you and the roughage will help your bowels!).

You need to switch off from the day's events and calm your mind. Allow plenty of time for your nightly routine. Have a warm bath or a good wash, clean your teeth, do a few relaxing exercises (we

have given you some on page 166), read a book or listen to the radio.
Many people do the newspaper crossword.

Sometimes it is just not possible to quieten our racing minds. We
go over and over the events of the day or the worries of tomorrow –
our thoughts get muddled and jumbled but still they will not stop.
We begin to get desperate about not getting to sleep, about being too
tired in the morning, and this increases our anxiety. This is when we
need to take more positive steps to help ourselves.

Quietening the Restless Mind

We either think orally using our tongue and throat muscles, literally
'talking' to ourselves, or we visualize using the muscles of our eyes.
In the latter case we watch our thoughts as if replaying or making a
film. Most people use both ways of thinking but usually rely on one
more than the other. If we need these muscles in order to think it is
clear that if we relax them completely, thinking will become impossible and we will be able to go to sleep.

To test this, lie down on the bed, place the fingertips of each hand
on either side of your throat so that you are able to feel your vocal
chords. Say out loud, 'Jack and Jill went up the hill . . .' (any such
nonsense will do!). Now whisper it to yourself feeling the muscles at
work – now say it to yourself without letting a muscle flicker. You
will find it almost impossible unless you start to visualize the pic-
tures. As we have seen before you can learn to release the tension in
these muscles by clenching the teeth and jaw and then relaxing,
letting the mouth fall loose and the tongue lie back.

Now test your eyes – again lying flat, close the lids and concentrate.
Imagine a room you know well and put three people in it. Now look
at the ceiling, the floor, the door, the window and the furniture; look
at the first person, the second person and then the third person. Do
the same routine but faster. You will feel your eyes moving round the
room. Now concentrate on one person in that room. Do not move
your eyes at all, but think of the ceiling, the floor, the door, the
window, and the furniture, the first person, the second person and
now the person at whom you are looking. Do that again faster but
do not move your eyes. If you do it properly it will be quite impossible.

Practise it regularly and you will be able to switch off your thoughts and drop off to sleep.

So, if you feel yourself getting into this groove of restless thinking, take action. Get out of bed, go downstairs and start again. If necessary get yourself something to eat or drink. Make sure you are warm and comfortable and then concentrate on releasing tension in those muscles. First in your jaw and neck – tense and relax several times to make sure it is really unwound. Secondly choose something to look at – a place you find restful, a favourite view, a childhood memory, look around and then concentrate on one thing. Focus your eyes on one thing only. You will soon fall asleep.

Rest is essential

Too often we meet members of our groups who resist taking a break during the day as they fear it will leave them not tired enough to go to sleep. It is much more likely that being overtired will have this effect. The more pressure you are under, the more important it is to plan some form of retreat and enforced idleness into your day. Do not limit your moments of relaxation to our 15-minute relaxation programme. Take every opportunity that presents itself – that wait in the supermarket queue, the ride in the bus, the time in the bath, use these minutes for positive relaxation: they can prepare you for hours of hard work and encourage sound sleep from which you will wake refreshed.

Thoughts to help perspective

To relax you need to master time and not be its slave. Take time and make use of it to care for yourself.

You need time to keep yourself fit and tough enough for your chosen lifestyle: exercise, nutrition and relaxation all need time.

Take time for recreation – hobbies are important, not only is changing your activity relaxing for mind and body, it is through these lateral interests we can learn to expand and create new dimensions in ourselves. Use all the time allotted to you for holidays – these recharge the batteries and recover the equilibrium.

Take major events one at a time when you can – moving house, getting married, having children, changing jobs, redundancy, conflicts, divorce, retirement, bereavement and many others – are momentous happenings and a considerable energy drain.

Take time to talk over any problems – just listening to yourself speaking about them can get your thoughts into perspective.

Take time to listen to others and try not to interrupt – their experience and advice may well be a help.

If things get out of hand – take time to consult your doctor. There is no disgrace in asking for help.

Part IV
Fitness in Sickness and in Health

This part of the book is about caring – for ourselves and for others. Chapter 7 encourages you to care for those parts of the body which show – the skin, hands and feet. It is no good having a well-fed, fully exercised, tension-controlled body if the outward appearance is neglected.

Chapter 8 deals with caring for yourself and others throughout life. At every stage of life our bodies have different needs, and we inevitably encounter problems and hazards. Although most of these have been recognized by generations and the answers are often common sense, it is easy to be caught unaware or unprepared. Knowledge and understanding of the facts can be invaluable when facing and surviving the challenges of each life stage.

Chapter 9 tackles preventive measures which can be taken to avoid illness and gives common sense advice on recurring ailments.

Chapter 10 discusses first aid. So many lives could be saved both in the home and outside by quick reactions and a basic knowledge of first aid, that we hope that everyone will not only read but constantly refer to this chapter and preferably take a professional course as well.

Chapter 7
Take Care of Yourself Day by Day

Skin

The skin makes up about 16 per cent of the total body weight and varies in thickness from 1 mm on the eyelids to 3 mm between the shoulder blades and on the palms of the hands and soles of the feet (though it can increase to 1 cm on the soles of those who habitually go around barefoot). There can be up to 20 sq. ft of skin on the body and its condition reflects age, habits, health, nutrition, heredity and lifestyle. The skin of fit people has a bloom no amount of artifice can achieve.

The skin is formed of two layers. The *dermis* or lower layer contains the nerves and fat cells, blood and lymph vessels, and from it emerge the sweat glands, sebaceous glands and hair follicles. Germs from outside the body do not reach the dermis unless the skin is damaged or diseased. It is protected by the *epidermis* or visible layer of our skin. Skin cells produced at the base of the epidermis push up towards the surface. This can take from 40 to 56 days and by the time the cell has reached the surface it has died. Every 24 hours each one of us peels off about 10,000 million of these skin scales (house dust is said to consist of 90 per cent dead skin!).

The skin has a surface barrier called an 'acid mantle' (made up of sebum and sweat). This protects the skin from bacteria and also effectively restricts the moisture in either direction.

Skin care starts with nutrition. A smooth skin needs healthy cell reproduction and for this it needs vitamins, minerals, proteins, fats and carbohydrates – all the nutrients that are essential to health. Fatty tissue is beneath the dermis in the subcutaneous layer so that a crash diet resulting in sudden weight loss or a diet entirely free from fat will result in loss of fat from this layer and the skin will look wrinkled and sagging.

Through the pores of our skin the body both 'breathes' and

excretes waste products. The process is vital for a healthy skin so it is essential to keep it free from pore-clogging grime.

Many doctors advocate the use of soap and water as being the best for cleaning the skin. However, central heating, pollution, climatic conditions and hard water all take their toll from the skin, diminishing its natural oils, and beauticians believe that we can help ourselves by replacing these with skin foods and moisturizers. Furthermore they feel that it is better to start using creams to clean and feed the skin at an early age rather than cry over the dryness and wrinkles later on! Certainly the skin foods keep the skin supple and soft and make-up can be cleverly and discreetly used to highlight the good points and play down those we wish to hide. Make-up is not only for fun and vanity, it also acts as a protection against all the dirt in the air.

Soap and water will not be sufficient however to remove make-up because of the oils used as a basis for the creams. This needs cleansing cream applied with an upward movement of the hand which will massage the face as well as cleanse the pores. There are so many different kinds of cosmetics on the market that it is difficult to know which one to choose. It is usually wiser to stick to one brand at a time as the colours and perfumes are often produced to complement each other. With a sensitive skin avoid any highly perfumed preparations as it is usually these which cause skin irritations and rashes. The bland varieties are often cheaper too!

Some skins need protection from the sun and there are now several products on the market which will screen out ultra-violet rays. For most of us sunbathing is a wonderful source of vitamin D and certainly a tanned skin not only gives a healthy appearance, it makes one feel good too. However, too much exposure to the sun will dry the skin until it becomes like leather. Make sure to keep the skin well oiled. Constant exposure of fair skinned people to sunlight in hot countries can lead to skin cancer.

Skin is sensitive to touch and indeed the body surface is so sensitive as to make gentle contact in almost any region a potentially sexual experience.

Body Odour

The skin is sensitive to changes in temperature. It helps in the regulation of body temperature by conserving or dissipating heat by the evaporation of sweat. An adult has in the region of 460 sweat glands per sq. in. (70 per sq. cm) on his back and over 2,600 per sq. in. (400 per sq. cm) on his palms and soles. Much of our water loss is through these sweat glands.

The salty fluid excreted by the glands is not in itself odorous, but the bacterial action on the sweat produces the scent with which, like animals, humans attract the opposite sex. The hair under our arm-pits and around the groin acts as a scent trap to retain the odours and intensify them. Shaving this hair reduces the odour. Why should humans, unlike other animals try to rid themselves of one of their most natural attractions by removing this hair, using deodorants and anti-perspirants, and masking natural smells with perfumes? The answer probably lies in the clothes we wear. One is not usually aware of the smell of sweat, but when it is trapped by our clothes and com-bined with overheated temperatures, dirt and pollution, bacteria can develop rapidly in the stale sweat and this produces a particularly abhorrent smell. Anyone who has taught in school will know that the 'smelly' child is ostracized, likewise the office or factory-worker with B.O. can become a social outcast. This can produce a nervous reaction in the sufferer which in turn brings on more sweating and exacerbates the problem. Unfortunately the whole situation becomes very embarrassing and the natural instinct seems to be to shy away rather than try to help. However, with tact, a lot can be done to ease the situation.

Obviously if the sufferer is a young schoolchild an approach should be made by the teacher or school doctor to the parents. Fresh under-clothing and discreet attention to hygiene for the child at school may be the answer. Care will have to be taken that the child does not become the butt for cruel remarks from his peers. The easiest and most natural place to deal with B.O. is within the home. In all cases it is essential that B.O. sufferers should not feel rejected. They must be made to feel that it is because they are wanted that the situation must be dealt with not because they themselves are disliked. It may be less embarrassing for everyone concerned if it is tackled by

N.P.S. – 12

someone in authority or 'uniform' such as a works' nurse or a medical officer.

Skin experts feel that repeated washing and clean clothes should be enough to prevent body odour and that chemical deodorants are an unnecessary and potentially damaging addition. However, generally deodorants are harmless (a few people are sensitive to them resulting in skin rashes) and they do mask B.O. Anti-perspirants are different and should only be used on very special occasions. These prevent the sweat glands from excreting and sometimes the glands can swell or infection become trapped and result in boils, usually in the hair follicles.

Everyone should change their underclothing every day. Once stale sweat has impregnated clothes it is impossible to wash away the smells. To conquer a B.O. problem, choose light cool clothes of natural materials, loosely fitted under the arm. Do not wear tight belts. Women have to be particularly careful during their monthly period or when breast feeding. Vaginal deodorants should never be necessary and should not be used as they can be dangerous.

Sweaty feet are usually a male problem and this can be especially bad during the teenage years when the glands may sweat profusely. Again clean socks and plenty of washing is usually the answer. Avoid man-made fibres, dry the feet well and use talcum powder if necessary. Track shoes, running and gym shoes should only be worn for their specific purpose as these do not allow the feet to 'breathe'. Ordinary shoes made of man-made fibre can be a problem too but shoe leather is expensive; this can be helped by using deodorizing inner soles. Change shoes frequently and allow them to air.

If sweating is very severe there is an operation which removes areas of skin and the maximum content of the sweat glands from the armpits. The major operation for hands and feet may have unwanted side effects and is not undertaken lightly.

Halitosis (Bad Breath)

Everyone suffers occasionally from smelly breath caused by eating strong foods such as garlic, onions or curry. This can be quite nauseous to others but they may be oblivious of it if they have eaten the same foods themselves. Stale smoke on the breath of smokers can have the same effect. In these cases the use of a mouth deodorant is usually quite sufficient.

A common cause is bad teeth. Poor general health or illness can also be indicated. If this is suspected visit your doctor or dentist. Bad breath can be a warning that something is wrong so do not ignore it.

Bad breath can also be caused by slimming! With a wholly high-protein diet, the smell on the breath is caused by the break down of the fat cells. This is one of the reasons it is important to include fresh fruit and vegetables in the diet. The other is to avoid constipation which is in itself a cause of halitosis.

Hair

An average scalp contains any number from 100 to 150,000 hairs! Each hair follicle is able to make three or more different kinds of hair. The first to appear is lanugo, the colourless silky soft hair sometimes seen on premature babies. This is usually superseded by vellus hair a month or two before birth. This type of hair remains throughout adulthood on our upper cheeks, ears, most of our bodies and limbs. It is often colourless and rarely grows longer than an inch. The hairs of the scalp, eyebrows and eyelashes are in contrast much coarser and more pigmented and in the case of our scalp much longer. This coarser hair and the hair which comes with puberty in the armpits, groin and on the chest is called terminal hair.

Hair follicles do not increase in number with age so the density of hair on a child is higher than that of an adult. Each follicle goes through a cycle of activity. The cycle of hair growth followed by withering and a rest period when no hair is produced is necessary to restrict the length of the shorter hairs and to replace damaged hair. The life of a vellus hair is about $4\frac{1}{2}$ months, while scalp hair lives for 3 to 5 years. It would take 6 years before becoming long enough to sit on and rarely grows longer than a metre.

Hair loss is determined by sex and heredity. Fifty-eight per cent of men will be substantially bald by the age of 50. One in five is very bald by 30! Women only occasionally go bald although they do lose some of their hair, particularly after childbirth or as a side-effect of the oral contraceptive pill. There is also a rare type of baldness which is caused by stress and often rights itself spontaneously.

Hair is dead and once damaged it can never repair itself. The first rule for looking after hair is to keep it clean and to trim it regularly. Choose an acid-balanced shampoo as this will not strip the hair of its own natural oils or damage it in any way (ask your chemist or hairdresser for advice). Change the shampoo occasionally as the hair will become resistant to one kind. Before washing the hair, give it a good brush. This will loosen the dirt and debris and also the dead skin cells. It will stimulate the scalp circulation too. (That is the reason Granny made a rule of 100 strokes of the brush a day!) It is much easier to use a shower spray to rinse the shampoo out of your hair. With dry and brittle or very fine hair a conditioner will give it body and bounce. Avoid using hair sprays. They simply glue individual hairs together where they cross and in spite of claims that they brush out, sprays inevitably leave a residue on the uneven surface of hair. Never backcomb hair and do not neglect to clean brushes and combs.

Hair colour and type, thick or thin, curly or straight, varies amazingly from race to race, but for everyone the best conditioner is the same – good health! Good nutrition and excellent circulation stimulated by exercise all contribute to make the hair a natural crowning glory.

Teeth

Oral hygiene and good diet are absolutely essential to keep teeth healthy and free from decay. A diet that is good for you is good for your teeth. Sugar and sticky foods lead to dental decay and inflamed gums. Pregnant women and children need foods containing calcium. Once teeth have formed, extra calcium does not help.

The enemy of teeth is plaque, which is a transparent scum of bacteria and enzymes from the saliva which clings to the teeth. When eating or drinking sugary foods, germs in the plaque turn these foods into acids which eat away the enamel covering of the teeth, causing decay. If not removed each day the plaque collects, becomes very hard to remove and irritates the gum.

For a healthy mouth it is better to get into the habit of brushing the teeth and gums in the morning after breakfast and at bed times. Rinse the mouth out with cold water after other meals. When brushing the teeth remember to use an anti-plaque toothbrush (i.e.

medium grade) with a small head and straight handle, and preferably a toothpaste containing fluoride as this has been shown to
protect teeth against decay. Correct brushing takes at least 3 minutes.
Remember to brush the upper and lower teeth, particularly the
inside, as well as the grinding or biting surfaces. Brush every surface
three times up and down and always start in the same place in your
mouth and do it the same way – then none will be neglected. The use
of dental floss is also necessary to remove plaque from areas where
the brush cannot reach. A word of warning: although the single most
effective way of counteracting the effects of a modern-day diet on
our teeth is a thorough brush at least once a day, hard brushes and
coarse paste can cause even more damage scratching the enamel like
scouring powders score the sides of a bath. These scratches allow
bacteria to penetrate and do further harm.

Visit the dentist regularly; see him as often as he advises, to have
teeth professionally cleaned and checked for cavities.

Eyes

Sparkling eyes are the gift of health and happiness. Nevertheless
even healthy eyes get tired occasionally and then they should be
rested under pads of damp cottonwool or lint. Screwing up the eyes
against brilliant sunshine encourages wrinkles and makes the eyes
sore. Protect them by wearing Polaroid sunglasses.

It is sound practice to get your eyes tested about every two years –
and have the glasses changed if necessary. Do not be afraid to change
the frames too – they can be a marvellous aid to good looks, and a
new shape may give both the wearer and the onlooker a new outlook!

Ears

The glands in the ear are modified to produce earwax. Dirty ears are
unsightly and the wax in the outer ear can become infected by the
bacteria which are normally harmless colonizers of the ear. As one
becomes older this wax can build up and become a solid plug effectively blocking the sound waves. It is easy for the doctor to remove it.

Hands and Nails

Protect the hands by wearing gloves when washing, gardening or cleaning the car. At the very least remember to use a barrier or hand cream before you start. Rough calloused hands are unattractive. If for any reason you have dirt deeply ingrained into the lines of your hands, mix equal quantities of oil and caster sugar and rub this into the palms and fingers. The oil will soften the skin and the sugar will collect the dirt.

Make sure your diet contains enough calcium for your nails. They need constant renewal. They also need regular cleaning as well as cutting or filing. Bitten nails not only look unsightly, they are also unhygienic.

Take Care of Yourself on Holiday

The trouble with holidays is that the planning is all in the mind and the exposition is carried out by the body! Holidays are like honeymoons, we often expect too much of them and of ourselves! It is all very well climbing a mountain in the mind's eye but it is quite a different matter to try to take a rotund, underexercised, probably ill-equipped body up a real path.

Plan your holiday with yourself in mind not the person you would like to be! It is no good planning to take your son for a walking holiday in the Lakes, harking back to the days of your prime, if you are now hopelessly out of condition and practice. It is not a good idea to plan to go camping if you cannot stand creepy-crawlies and have had enough of washing up. You must decide if you are the sort of person who needs the stimulation of sight-seeing or if you can switch off and lie in the sun all day. Do you need as well as want to be energetic or lazy? If you are going on holiday with the family, there are many holidays which enable everyone to 'do their own thing'.

Plan to be fit enough to enjoy your holiday. Many people work long hours either doing overtime to earn extra cash or finishing up their work in order to go away. By the time the day of the holiday arrives they are completely exhausted. We would like to suggest that you try one of our fitness courses (see page 246) seriously for six weeks prior to your holiday so that you are in excellent condition to enjoy it.

Plan to be slim enough to put on just a little weight. One of the chief joys of a holiday can be the food. If you are slim enough to have a few pounds in hand you can increase your intake with a free conscience. Remember to take it slowly at first – you will probably not be used to such a rich and liberal diet. You do not want to end up with an upset stomach.

Plan to go slowly at first. Too many people throw themselves into their holiday with abandoned zeal – they swim, run around the beach, surf, sail, walk, climb and then dance all night. Five days into the holiday and they cannot understand the lethargy which descends on them. They are tired out. Occasionally it is worse than that – the hospitals near holiday centres are quite used to the holiday heart attacks and the unnecessary broken legs. Read the obituary columns, too many deaths occur on holiday!

Plan to take the right gear. Find out all you can about the sort of holiday you are planning to take and make sure you have the right equipment. There are far too many accidents because holiday-makers are ill-prepared – walking with gym shoes, sailing without lifejackets, lazing in rubber dinghies without being able to swim, no skin oil for the sun, no gloves for the cold. Do not forget to have the relevant injections if you are going abroad. Make sure you are covered by medical insurance and remember that if you are pregnant this often needs separate cover.

Have a good time!

Take Care of Yourself in Extremes

Normally human bodies are well equipped to deal with changes of temperature but there are some rules it makes sense to keep.

In the cold

Eat a good nourishing diet (it does not necessarily have to be hot food) to give enough energy to combat the weather. Several layers of light clothing are warmer than one heavy overcoat and it is most important to keep the extremities covered and wind- and water-proofed. Take plenty of exercise to keep the circulation flowing.

Extreme cold can be dangerous to young babies and old people. Hypothermia is commonly referred to as 'deadly cold'. The very young and very old have more difficulty in maintaining body heat because their circulation is not efficient and they cannot move around easily. Hundreds and perhaps thousands of deaths could be prevented every year if only people realized the danger. The sufferer from this complaint will become drowsy and very ill quite rapidly; their skin will feel icy to the touch. It is very important not to warm them up too quickly (do *not* use hot water bottles or electric blankets) as this will increase the danger – get them to the hospital without delay.

In a heatwave

Wear light, loose clothing of natural fibres. If possible, it makes sense to revise a living pattern, waking early, having a siesta in the afternoon and then working again in the cool of the evening. Eat plenty of light meals with fresh fruit and salad, drink as much fluid as you can (but remember the calories – excess weight does not help you keep cool!). If the heat is really exceptional, salt tablets may help.

Too much sun is not good for the skin but people cannot resist sunbathing. If you overdo it and suffer from sunburn you will find that calamine lotion, talcum powder and even cold water will have a soothing effect. Drink plenty of cold fluids to prevent dehydration.

In very hot weather the effects of the heat can be quite dangerous. Heat exhaustion can result from excessive sweating when working under hot conditions. The loss of salt and water from the body results in complete exhaustion, the skin is pale and moist and the temperature may be a little raised. Cool surroundings and a drink of water with salt ($\frac{1}{4}$ teaspoon of salt to each $\frac{1}{2}$ pint, or 2·8 dl, of water) may well help. *Heat or sun stroke* is quite another matter. In this case the body is unable to lose the excess heat and the skin is flushed, dry and burning to the touch. The temperature is very high and the person may lose consciousness. In this case it is important to get medical aid very urgently. Meanwhile remove all clothes and cover the body with a wet sheet and sprinkle with water. Either fan by hand or get an electric fan.

Chapter 8
Take Care of Yourself and
Others Throughout Life

There are times in our lives when sheer determination is not enough to attain or maintain an acceptable level of fitness. At certain periods of hormone change, growing up or ageing, an intelligent informed approach can minimize difficulties or even prevent serious trouble.

The Menstrual Cycle

Sometime between the ages of 10 and 17, although more usually between 12 and 14, a small girl's figure slowly begins to develop into that of a young woman, with breasts, hips and the growth of hair both under her arms and in the pubic region. Shortly after this she will probably notice a little blood staining from her vagina and this will be her first period. Some girls go straight into a regular 28 days' cycle but many others have one period and then miss several months before they have another. After a year or two the periods should settle down to a regular cycle but one in three girls are still not regular by the age of 17.

Every woman varies in the amount of blood she loses at each period. Some women lose only slightly for one or two days, while others lose heavily for seven or eight days. Both are quite normal and have no bearing on the ability to conceive. Periods are not an illness but a normal part of a healthy woman's bodily function. Normally there is nothing to be gained by altering your day-to-day activities when you are menstruating. It is, however, essential to take extra care of your personal hygiene and the cleanliness of your underclothing.

The most common cause of missed periods is pregnancy. Periods can also be missed at times of extra excitement or strain such as starting a new job or going to college. It can also occasionally be the result of jet travel because of sudden time changes. If, however, after the periods have settled down into a regular monthly cycle you miss more than two consecutive periods it would be sensible to consult your doctor. As is shown by those suffering from anorexia nervosa, rapid dieting can also be a cause of missed periods.

Dysmenorrhoea (Painful Periods)

The majority of women have slight discomfort with menstruation but at least 45 per cent of women experience strong pain. It can be incapacitating and affect social life and personal relationships. Many women lose time at work during the first two menstrual days and it is probably the biggest single medical problem in adolescent girls. It is estimated that 140 million work hours a year are lost in America because of dysmenorrhoea. There is also a pain which is occasionally experienced at the mid-menstrual period, without any effusion of blood. This is called Mittelschmerth.

However, help is at hand. As one doctor puts it, 'Although the assumption that man is born to suffer and women are born to suffer more than man is still held by many to be true, it need not be so for dysmenorrhoea; for we can relieve pain and suffering in the majority of women.'

1. Primary dysmenorrhoea

This affects young women, often beginning within one or two years of the onset of menstruation, it becomes less severe at 25 to 30 years of age or after pregnancy. There are two types and both can be relieved:

Congestive dysmenorrhoea occurs just before and for the first day or two of the period. There may be an engorged, bloated feeling and the lower part of the tummy and the breasts may feel tender. This is mainly due to the salt and water build-up in the body. The pain is dull and aching and may be accompanied by a headache and backache. You can help yourself by taking a suitable analgesic (consult your chemist about this), making sure you are not constipated and taking a little extra exercise. You will find the exercises on page 189, Fig. 22, will help you.

Spasmodic dysmenorrhoea is shorter in duration and usually occurs on the first day of a period. The pain is low down in the pelvis and is colicky in nature. The treatment here is to curl up with a hot water bottle for a few hours after taking an effective pain-killing tablet. Very few women need surgical help with this problem but occasionally a minor operation – a D and C (dilation and curettage) – may be necessary in the most severe cases.

2. Secondary dysmenorrhoea

This describes painful menstruation usually beginning in later life. This pain can build up before a period and is more a dull ache in quality than primary dysmenorrhoea. This can be the result of organic disease of the reproductive system such as fibroids or infections. This needs medical treatment and you should not hesitate to consult your doctor.

Premenstrual tension (Congestive Dysmenorrhoea)

The premenstrual syndrome is one of the civilized world's most common diseases. It can suddenly transform a happy-go-lucky woman into a tense, depressed, irritable and lethargic one as a result of the alterations in the levels of her menstrual hormones.

The 'paramenstruum' describes the four days before a period and the four days immediately after the beginning of the blood flow. Recent surveys have given incontrovertible evidence that this monthly event, quite apart from the discomfort to the woman herself, represents quite a hazard to the community at large. During these eight days women become mentally dull, more clumsy and accident-prone. Many prison admissions of women occur during this time. A large number of all women's emergency admissions to medical, surgical, accident, infectious fevers and psychiatric wards occur during the paramenstruum when there is lowered pain tolerance, lowered resistance to infection, and generalized fluid retention. There are also abnormal mental, physical and emotional responses to situations which are totally out of character with the individual. At this time of their cycle schoolgirls may find their mental ability impaired and from time to time their chance of passing examinations may be in jeopardy. They are also liable to receive more punishments for misdemeanours at this time, and indeed, school prefects administer more punishments while in their own paramenstruum. The sudden aggressive outbursts which can occur with premenstrual tension can often result in marital quarrels, irrational decisions, guilty feelings and perhaps the greatest tragedy of all – the battered baby. A man's work can be affected too by his partner's paramenstrual irritability.

Premenstrual tension only lasts a day or two for some women but there are others in whom the mood swing begins at ovulation and continues until menstruation, lasting sometimes for at least 2 weeks in each month. If the hormonal imbalance in your case is of short duration, it is probably only necessary for you to recognize it for what it is and arrange your most important engagements and assignments for your alert, vivacious postmenstrual phase. For some reason this premenstrual time seems to be accompanied by a loss of memory and you may need reminding of the reason why you are depressed, 'have no friends' or have a sudden craving for carbohydrates! A sympathetic mother, friend, lover or husband should be alerted to remember the date! It will help them too to understand that the cruel remarks, the odd behaviour, should not be taken personally. Try our exercises (see Fig. 22).

If, however, your life is considerably hampered by this disease it will give you heart to know that complete medical help is possible in most cases. Thanks largely to the work and research being done in Great Britain by Dr Katarina Dalton and her team and also St Thomas' Hospital, London, much human suffering and its consequences can be alleviated. In the past many women have tried valiantly and unsuccessfully to 'pull themselves together'.

Work already carried out by Dr Katarina Dalton strongly suggests that the progesterone-oestrogen balance is implicated in the premenstrual syndrome problem. In fact for some twenty years she has been treating P.M.S. with pure progesterone and claims a high degree of success. This treatment cannot be taken orally and is only available in the form of injections, pessaries and suppositories which are expensive and not always considered convenient to use.

Synthetic progesterone-like substances known as progestogens can be taken by mouth but to date have not proved to be successful. The combination birth control pill, containing progestogen, certainly worked for some women but for others actually induced a form of depression almost as bad as the P.M.S. it was supposed to be curing.

Premenstrual Tension

Starting position 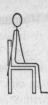 Fig. 22

Gently rub tummy in painful area and lower back. Do these exercises gently several times a day, at work, at home, on the loo. Breathe naturally throughout exercises. See Loo Exercises, also very good for premenstrual tension.

1. *Alternate knee bend*

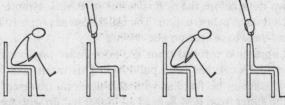

Bend one knee to chest – stretch arms above head and circle back to sides

2. *Pelvic tilting*

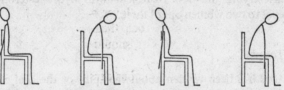

Arch and round spine. Head back and forwards. Roll back and forth on buttocks

3. *Lift alternate buttocks*

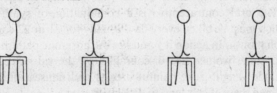

Rock from one buttock to the other

4. *Cross legs and tense abdominal muscles*

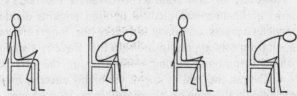

Tighten tummy muscles hard – lean forwards. Cross one leg over the other. Grasp both legs together hard

Recently, however, new work at St Thomas' Hospital in London, has shown that another synthetic progestogen, dydrogesterone gives relief from P.M.S. in around 70 per cent of cases. The chemical structure of this particular progestogen is very similar to that of pure progesterone which may account for its greater effectiveness. But it has also been used in a very special way, starting treatment from two days before the normal onset of P.M.S. symptoms right up to the time of menstruation. The usual dose has been 10 mg twice daily and there have been no side-effects.

Further controlled trials are now under way but meanwhile the original work has been published. This means that many doctors will already be familiar with this new oral treatment. Now women who suffer from P.M.S. need no longer put up with something which makes life miserable for themselves and their families, without at least trying the new treatment with dydrogesterone which gives relief to two women out of three.

'The pill'

More has been written about the 'pill' or the oral contraceptive in recent years than any other contraceptive method and many questions still remain unanswered.

The oral contraceptive is a combination of synthetic hormones which must be taken every day, usually for 21 or 22 consecutive days each month. In action it simulates the hormone pattern of pregnancy, and some women are discouraged by the side-effects, which may include weight-gain, painful breasts and nausea, although in most women these effects tend to disappear after a time.

However, all oral contraceptives affect the body's complicated hormone balance and medical opinion remains divided about the possible dangers of taking the drug for long periods. The latest medical reports appear to indicate that there is a slightly increased risk of thrombosis among women taking the oral contraceptive. Nevertheless, the 'pill' is one of the highly effective methods of contraception, although in absolute terms it does not provide the assurance of 100 per cent protection which is sometimes claimed. Research is continuing in an endeavour to develop an improved pill.

Sexual intercourse

Sexual enjoyment needs energy! Many a potentially successful couple have come to grief because of the temporary exhaustion of one of the two partners. It is pretty difficult to come home from a hard day's work, clean the flat with a flourish, whip up a little dinner for friends, entertain and then go to bed with one's partner with satisfaction on both sides, and rise with the lark the next morning to start the round again! Cleaning and cooking on their own can be very tiring indeed.

It is also underestimated how long it takes to get over childbirth, let alone how much coping with several babies takes out of a woman's strength. She also has to carry alone the worries and traumas of bringing up the babies and toddlers. All the time she is physically and mentally learning about childcare and coping in an unsympathetic world. No wonder that sometimes she is worn out and finds care of herself let alone physical demonstration towards her husband well-nigh impossible! Our Exercises with Partner (see Fig. 23) may help.

Men can be temporarily made impotent from exhaustion. They may appear to be a regular Casanova taking out (and presumably to bed) two or three different girls in a week – but they may feel quite daunted when faced with an ever ready opportunity night after night and day after day! They might too be using up most of their energy working on a new job or worrying over the bills. Maybe a bout of flu or some other illness has sapped their strength and they need time to recover.

Very often these causes of frigidity or failure can be overlooked and the partner feels personally affronted. Understanding talk between the couple can be a great help but when one or both of them are exhausted talking out the problem may not help at all. Tired minds do not know the truth and will often speak unselected and hurtful thoughts that are not meant at all. In the early years of a partnership or marriage it is wise to keep the health of the body at the forefront of your thoughts. Time will again help you to recognize signs of weariness in each other and teach you the patience to aid recovery.

For stamina and energy it is essential to eat well but wisely, taking regular exercise. Exercises together not only tone up the muscles but also teach you to explore each other's bodies. On page 192 (Fig. 23) are a series of exercises which can either be done together in a gym fully clothed or else naked in the privacy of the bedroom.

Exercises with Partner

Fig. 23

No movement takes place – muscle tightens and relaxes. Try to do movement but partner stops you. Keep breathing naturally throughout exercises.

Starting positions   Lying front and back

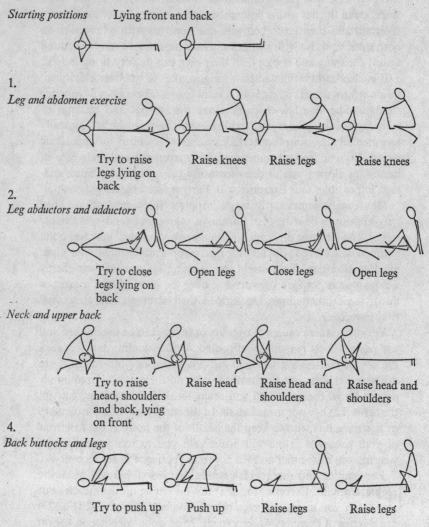

1.

Leg and abdomen exercise

| Try to raise legs lying on back | Raise knees | Raise legs | Raise knees |

2.

Leg abductors and adductors

| Try to close legs lying on back | Open legs | Close legs | Open legs |

Neck and upper back

| Try to raise head, shoulders and back, lying on front | Raise head | Raise head and shoulders | Raise head and shoulders |

4.

Back buttocks and legs

| Try to push up | Push up | Raise legs | Raise legs |

Pregnancy

It might be difficult to think of pregnancy as anything other than an endurance test during the first three months, but, from the fourth month onwards, the mother-to-be can feel and look her best. To help achieve this enviable state some rules must be observed.

Eating well but not for two

A pregnant mother needs extra nutrients but the total calorie intake should remain the same. The weight-gain over the 9 months' pregnancy should be in the region of 22 lb (10 kg) and no more.

The essential requirements for a healthy growth of the baby are vitamins A and D; calcium to form the baby's bones and teeth (a lack of adequate calcium in the diet often means that the growing baby uses up the calcium stores from the mother's own body, causing her serious tooth decay); iron to cope with the 25 per cent increase in the volume of the mother's blood; protein and of course the other main vitamins and minerals. The foods which supply these are milk (at least one pint a day should be drunk during pregnancy), cheese, meat and offal (particularly liver and kidney), fish (especially oily fish such as herrings, kippers and sardines which supply vitamin D and calcium), fruit and vegetables and wholemeal flour to provide adequate roughage to help prevent constipation. Apart from the generous milk allowance, these foods would all be found in a good slimming diet. You should still avoid refined starches and sugary foods. They will only increase your body fat without giving any nourishment to the baby.

Cravings

With any luck the longing will be for grapefruit, kippers, strawberries or curry. During pregnancy, as well as during differing phases of the menstrual cycle, a woman's taste sense is blunted and the need may be for something really tasty. However, if it's cream buns or jam doughnuts make sure it is not an excuse for self-indulgence! Occasionally a mother-to-be has a passion for something quite bizarre such as coal, clay, or even soap. Provided it is not poisonous or fattening it will probably do no harm but check with your clinic just to make sure!

Smoking

This is never good for the health. However, smoking during pregnancy can be lethal. It doubles the risk of miscarriage and increases the health risks to the baby. To go on smoking while you are carrying the baby means that you are deliberately increasing his chances of being born underweight and being more vulnerable to ill-health. Every pregnant woman should give up smoking – take this opportunity of giving up this harmful habit now you have a double incentive.

Plenty of exercise

It is necessary to keep the muscles in good working order not only for the hard work of the birth itself but also for getting the figure quickly back into shape afterwards. Walk everywhere. Swimming too is an ideal form of exercise – the water will support the extra weight and tones up your muscles.

Many of our Slimnastics group members who become pregnant continue to attend classes until about the last six weeks. They do as many of the exercises as they can leaving out the ones that become uncomfortable or in some cases impossible. The regular weight check helps to keep their weight under control and the group support is refreshing and relaxing. We encourage our young mums to attend the ante-natal classes for the last six weeks. This gives them a chance to meet other mothers-to-be from the same area and to get to know the hospital staff and routines. They can then rejoin our Mother and Child groups about six weeks after the birth.

Care of the back

As already mentioned in Chapter 1, pregnant and nursing mothers are among those most 'at risk' to back pain and injury. In order to facilitate the growth and birth of the baby, hormones act on the joints and the spine to make them more supple and lax. The extra weight of the baby causes postural strain and the stretching of the abdominal and pelvic muscles leads to a weakening of spinal support both in pregnancy and afterwards. This combination of lax spinal joints and weak abdominal muscles predisposes a young mother to mechanical injury even from such simple tasks as lifting up the baby from the cot. This means taking even more care than usual when lifting or carrying. Avoid picking up anything from floor level. With another toddler who inevitably begs to be carried, either sit down and encourage him to clamber on to the knee first for a little cuddle or else get him to climb on to the chair and pick him up off that.

Relaxation and enough rest

However busy the life, whether still working at a job or looking after other toddlers, remember that the body is already working overtime, not only living but creating. This is one time in life when it is perfectly justified to take time off to read, to sunbathe or to listen to the radio. That puritan urge which makes us think we must be seen to be busy can be kept at bay by the knowledge that the pregnant body is physically at work 24 hours of the day! Practise the tension control techniques. They are not only very useful during the birth but invaluable afterwards.

Attending the clinic regularly

They will monitor the progress of both you and your baby and spot any potential difficulties, and they will also help you with any problems or anxieties you may have. The clinic will supply you with extra vitamins and iron tablets. Iron pills can cause constipation, and if this is the case, ask the clinic to change them for another prescription.

Post-natal

After the birth

Breast feeding gives the very best nutritional start to the baby. About 8 lb (3·6 kg) of the weight gained during pregnancy is actual body fat in the mother and this forms a natural reserve of fat to be used during breast feeding. This reserve is necessary because with the average human milk production being almost 2 pints (1 litre) a day it requires an extra 1,000 calories a day in terms of body fuel. What you must not forget is that it is this reserve that is providing these calories and so you have no need to eat those extra calories each day if you are breast feeding your baby. Plenty of fluid is needed and this means *water* – not a food like milk as this adds on the extra calories which will only be retained as fat. So does the stout and red wine so beloved by the 'old wives' – we rather suspect that this was valued for its soporific effect on both mother and baby!

Breast feeding stimulates a contraction of the body tissues so – aided by a good supporting bra, which will prevent the weight dragging down from the upper chest – it actually improves the mother's figure. If breast feeding is impossible it is essential to concentrate on the chest exercises (see Fig. 10 on page 52) to strengthen the muscles supporting the bustline. Combine these with a strict low calorie diet in order to regain a pre-pregnancy shape.

Exercises are essential

The physiotherapists give some exercises to do in hospital after the birth of the baby. Unfortunately we know only too well that once at home it is only too easy to let good intentions remain just that! It is however, very, very important to take time off to concentrate on getting the body back into shape both externally and internally. As so many mothers come out of hospital as early as 48 hours after the birth we give exercises to be done from the second day onwards (see Fig. 24). Do these regularly and they will not only help now, they will save a lot of trouble in the future (prolapses, bowel trouble, back pain – all these can stem from an untoned pelvic floor). Remember to check the posture constantly. It is a temptation to go on standing as if still 'carrying all before you' (see Fig. 5, page 39).

Take plenty of rest

It is the six weeks after the birth that the mother really needs cherishing but it is often a very busy disheartening time. Suddenly all the attention is diverted to the baby and a lot is expected of the rather tired and maybe even inexperienced mother. It takes a whole six weeks for the hormonal balance to return to normal and during this

Post-natal Exercises

Fig. 24

Repeat 2–3 times a day – do each exercise 6 times slowly, at one go.

DO NOT HOLD YOUR BREATH

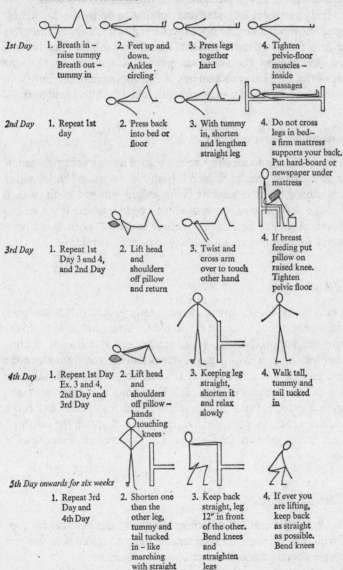

1st Day
1. Breath in – raise tummy Breath out – tummy in
2. Feet up and down. Ankles circling
3. Press legs together hard
4. Tighten pelvic-floor muscles – inside passages

2nd Day
1. Repeat 1st day
2. Press back into bed or floor
3. With tummy in, shorten and lengthen straight leg
4. Do not cross legs in bed – a firm mattress supports your back. Put hard-board or newspaper under mattress

3rd Day
1. Repeat 1st Day 3 and 4, and 2nd Day
2. Lift head and shoulders off pillow and return
3. Twist and cross arm over to touch other hand
4. If breast feeding put pillow on raised knee. Tighten pelvic floor

4th Day
1. Repeat 1st Day Ex. 3 and 4, 2nd Day and 3rd Day
2. Lift head and shoulders off pillow – hands touching knees
3. Keeping leg straight, shorten it and relax slowly
4. Walk tall, tummy and tail tucked in

5th Day onwards for six weeks
1. Repeat 3rd Day and 4th Day
2. Shorten one then the other leg, tummy and tail tucked in – like marching with straight legs
3. Keep back straight, leg 12" in front of the other. Bend knees and straighten legs
4. If ever you are lifting, keep back as straight as possible. Bend knees

time not only is the body not at its best or most attractive, with hair and skin likely to suffer and the back at its most vulnerable, emotions are probably all topsy-turvy too. It is important to remember that this phase will pass even though it feels like a lifetime. It is the result of the body getting re-adjusted and nothing to do with being unable to cope. The mother should not expect too much of herself and every bit of help that is offered, whether it be from husband, neighbours, relatives or friends, should be accepted. Do not believe all those stories of the mothers who leap out of bed coping magnificently with baby, toddlers, husband and household. It is they who are abnormal!

Get your weight under control

It is very important to lose any weight gained during your pregnancy. Some of the most serious cases of obesity in women of childbearing age are caused by extra pounds being gained with the birth of each child. If the next pregnancy starts with a weight problem it is a serious disadvantage and complications such as toxaemia, high blood pressure and a long labour are more likely to be experienced.

Join a group

Most people no longer live in large family groups when mothers, grandmothers, aunts, uncles et al. shared the strain of bringing up the younger generation. Nowadays we really need our friends. Young mothers with similar problems, anxieties and interests can share the burdens and the joys; they can organize a baby-sitting circle, arrange outings or help in times of need. The local church or clinic may well run such a group, if not, get together with a few friends and run a Slimnastics group in your own home. You will get all the information you need on this in Chapter 12, Courses of Exercises for Groups.

Go on attending the clinic

This is very important not only for the baby's sake but also for you. They will keep a check on your health too and make sure you are getting the added vitamins and iron you may need.

Babies

We still have not quite got away from the feeling that a fat baby is a 'bonny' one! This is of course totally untrue. An overweight baby is more prone to chest, lung and respiratory infections. But many young mothers still feel that a rapid weight-gain in the first few months is important. As a rough guide the baby should gain about half a pound (227 g) a week after the first fortnight of life. However, it is wise to check this with the clinic. They usually have a weight/ length chart which gives a more accurate assessment than an age/weight ratio.

Solid foods are sometimes introduced too early, perhaps when a child is only one month old and then it may be some form of cereal. If the baby is doing quite well on milk (breast or bottle) it is not necessary to introduce any solids until 3 to 4 months at the earliest and then it should be a purée of vegetables or fruit. When you do gradually begin to give the baby these solid foods it is quite easy and much cheaper to purée small portions of the family food. In this way sugar can be kept to the minimum and the baby will grow accustomed to the way you cook and eat.

Massaging the baby

In hot climates mothers love to sit gently playing with their babies, massaging and exercising their limbs. We feel that this establishes a feeling of contact and pleasure for both mother and baby and could become a regular part of the day's routine. In a warm room, perhaps just after the baby's bath, listen to a tape or record of relaxing music, sit down on the bed or the floor, legs stretched out in front and back supported by the bedhead or wall; covering the lap with a plastic sheet and a thick towel, gently massage the baby with baby oil, doing the exercises described in Fig. 25.

Toddlers

'Mealtimes can be just as important for nourishing family life as well as our bodies', so says the British Nutrition Foundation leaflet, 'Healthy Eating for Your Children'. It is a great temptation to get

Mother and Baby

Fig. 25

Gentle massage and exercises are a great favourite in hot climates. Use baby oil, and massage the limbs and surfaces.

Starting position

 Towel   Mother sitting with thick towel over stretched-out legs.

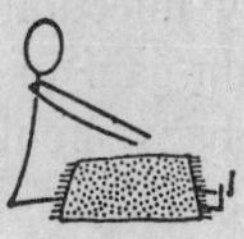

1. *Legs stretching and bending*

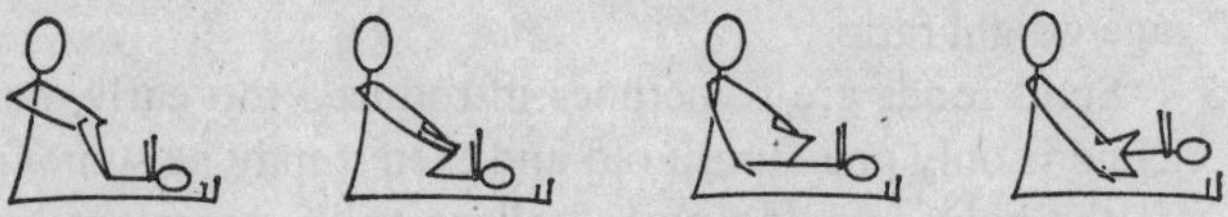

Leg exercises and massage with baby on back

2. *Arms stretching and bending*

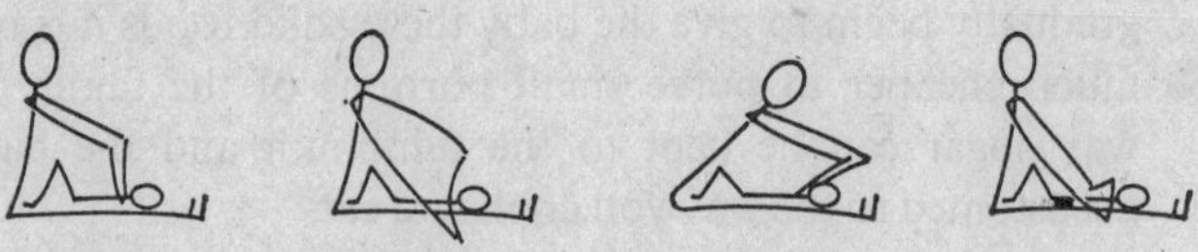

Arm exercises and massage with baby on back

3. *Back arch and flex*

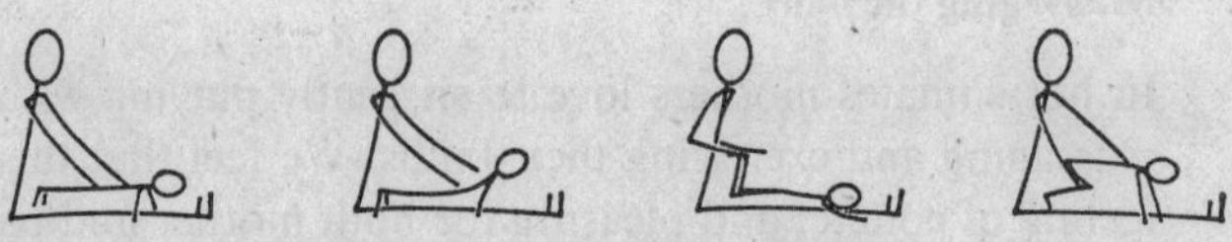

Massage back and under arms, feet etc. Let the baby do his own head lifting etc.

4. *Back and side arch and bend*

  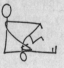 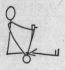

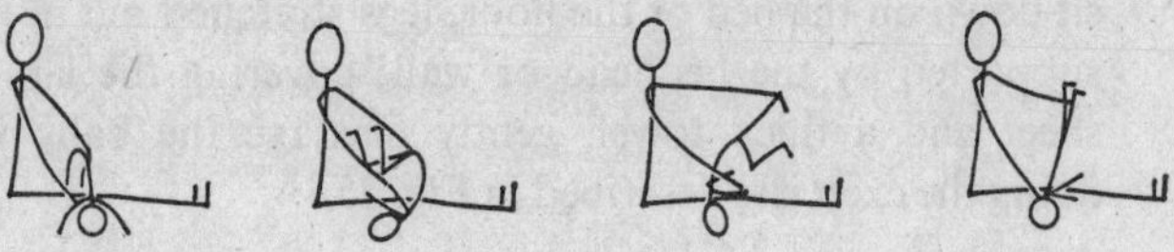

Massage back and sides. Place baby across lap and turn from side to side. Bend and stretch arms and legs together

into the habit of quick convenience foods on a tray in front of the T.V. (which is in all probability bombarding the young innocent with the joys of sweets, desserts and drinks without which no life is said to be complete!). If we care for our children at all this is a danger which should be avoided.

Good nutrition is a family affair and mealtimes should be social occasions not just hastily snatched snacks. It is important to establish good eating habits from the start; bad ones with their consequent weight problems tend to be passed down from generation to generation. The way to make sure that children pass on sound dietary principles to their children is to set them a good example, providing nutritious well-balanced meals in the home. As soon as they can, encourage them to help cook and prepare the food and from the start constantly teach them about how and what to eat.

The battle of wills

Almost overnight that sweet little baby can become the most infuriating little being! Suddenly from eating a wide variety of foods which have been carefully and lovingly prepared the toddler may decide to eat only a very small number of foods and refuse all others. It is very hard for the young mother to 'keep her cool' and take all this rejection in her stride. This is just the effect the toddler seems to be aiming for! The first thing is to realize that this is part of growing up. No healthy child will let himself starve and many of them need surprisingly little food. It is very important not to fight with a rebellious toddler over his food as this will lead to long-term problems and children usually survive this faddy phase remarkably well.

The most important foods for growing children who need plenty of energy are milk and dairy products, meat, fish, eggs, beans, wholemeal bread and other cereal foods. A daily pint of milk is a good way of making sure a child gets his daily nourishment but if this is his 'dislike' of the moment disguise it in cooking by making soups, jellies, puddings and sauces. Vegetables are frequently on the 'not wanted' list and the lack of essential vitamins and minerals may be a worry. To make sure a child does not suffer in any way it is a wise precaution to keep giving children under school age the vitamin preparations available from the clinic.

Don't be conned

It is very important not to be conned into buying peace from a child with sweets and snacks such as crisps and ice creams. These add few nutrients and many calories to the child's diet. Sweet foods should never be used as a comfort or reward. The association between love, comfort and sweet foods can set a dangerous pattern for the future – in moments of stress or celebration in adult life it is these foods which will seem attractive. It is equally unwise to ban these foods altogether. Forbidden excitements are far more tempting. Sweets should be for high-days and holidays only and at any other time the children should buy their own out of their pocket money. Of course example is the best deterrent!

Exercise for toddlers

This age group gets lots of exercise as they are exploring all the time. It is a good idea to get out in the open at least once a day. It gives an opportunity for both mother and child to let off steam and has a good chance of promoting a healthy appetite. Of course our Slimnastics Mother and Child groups are full of toddlers – most of the youngsters just potter around but quite a number join in the exercises too (see Fig. 26).

Children

Off to school

Breakfast is not only a nourishing start to the day, but children who have breakfast are more likely to be awake and alert at school and are less accident-prone than those who miss this meal. This is also true for adults. Breakfast does not have to be cooked or elaborate; there are good ideas in our recipe section. If the child comes down to the breakfast table in a really bad mood morning after morning he may need an early morning apple or glass of milk when woken and before getting out of bed. In many households this is the only meal at which the whole family meet during the weekday and it is a pity to spoil it

Fig. 26

Exercises to do together – for fun, relaxation, fitness and strength

1. Hold hands   Rock to and fro

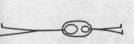 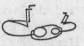

2. Hold hands   Bend knees   Stretch legs   Bend knees

  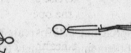

3. Gently   Bend child's legs   Both straighten and lie down   Up and bend

4. Slowly   Forwards to lying   Up to prone-kneeling   Back and squash thighs

with a surly face. Some children find it really impossible to eat early on in the morning and they should be given some fruit and a piece of cheese to eat in the playground.

Lunch

School meals vary drastically from one part of the country to another and although the recommended calorie value of a school lunch in the United Kingdom is 800 calories this could easily be made up of starchy foods. It might be much more satisfactory to give your child a packed lunch when you can be sure of giving him a well-balanced meal that you know he will enjoy and eat. Make things easy for yourself and buy a lunch box that fits in the school satchel and also can be kept overnight in the fridge. These lunches can be very attractive and nourishing and we give you plenty of ideas for these on page 122.

Coming home

Not only the children but also parents can hit an all-time low at tea-time and all of them might willingly tuck into doorstops of bread and jam, doughnuts and cream buns! Firm steps are needed to avoid falling into this trap. First thing, give the unruly mob an instant titbit such as a banana or other fruit or one piece of wholemeal toast with peanut butter or marmite (no more or they will lose their appetite); then make a large cup of tea or hot bouillon. Do not sit down but immediately set to work to make a high-tea for the children. Serve such supper dishes as spaghetti bolognese, macaroni cheese, cottage pie in winter and a variety of salads in the summer. Winter salads can be served alongside the hot dish instead of more cooked vegetables. Children love colour and a good variety attractively set out adds taste appeal. If you help the children to the food give them small amounts, they can always ask for more. As they grow older they should help themselves to the amount they need and then be expected to finish the plateful. Have a bowl of fruit always available for snacks.

After their bath and before bed children can have a cup of hot chocolate and perhaps one sweet biscuit. This sends them contentedly off to sleep. We find that this routine suits even much older children and students who come home tired from school and have several hours of homework or need to go out to clubs or sports training later in the evening.

The overweight child

Prevention is better than cure. When it is no longer possible to see a child's ribs it is time to stop the weight-gain before it gets too far. There is no such thing as 'puppy fat' and children do not usually grow out of being overweight without some positive aid in the form of dieting or increased exercise. Nor can the excess weight be put down to family tendencies; it is more likely the faulty eating habits the child has inherited rather than glandular problems.

Slimming a child is not easy because it draws more attention to his fatness about which he is probably already very self-conscious. A child is also still growing and needs to have enough of the right nutrients for his growing body, particularly at puberty. Therefore any diet should be undertaken with the supervision of a doctor.

The overweight child is probably only too willing to co-operate for he is often extremely unhappy about his weight and may well have to stand for much teasing at school. The eating pattern suggested above for the schoolchild makes it simple to monitor the calorie intake for all the meals and he will not seem different to his schoolmates. Visits to the tuck shop should be for low calorie chewing gum only and an extra glass of water at mealtimes will help to fill his stomach.

Emotionally, excess weight can be more disturbing to the adolescent girl than the adolescent boy, so it is important that the problem be controlled before puberty. An adolescent girl who is overweight may cut down drastically on the amount of food she eats and this can have very serious consequences, particularly in relation to glandular development and menstruation. To avoid this danger, an early pre-puberty weight checking programme is important.

Exercise is vital

Exercise is essential for children who are overweight, but most of us do not get enough exercise. It used to be considered usual for a seven-year-old to walk two to three miles to school, but now the car or a bus is the rule. Swimming, games of football and long walks will be extremely good for the whole family.

Teenagers

The teenage girl and her figure

The majority of adolescent girls wish to be less fat. Of course they are not all too fat by any manner of means but with puberty they naturally gain the fat of the hips and the breasts of the maturing female body. Unfortunately for some time the media have promoted the tall, skinny asexual teenager as the desirable 'norm' and for many girls this has been their unattainable goal. Just when they are told they should be having the best times of their lives they find themselves spotty, lumpy, grumpy, tired and overworked!

The best asset which a girl can have at this time is a good grounding in nutrition and biology of her own body. This will not only have helped her to keep her weight under control before puberty but also to understand that this mixed-up period of her life will soon pass. Cutting down the fats and the sugar in her diet will help the skin not to be too affected by the hormone changes; plenty of fruit and vegetables will add the vitamins and roughage which is very necessary at this time. Protein is important too to help build this mature body, and of course foods containing iron are necessary when the periods begin.

Without a good grounding in these facts of life some girls can become very unhappy indeed during this phase of their development. If they have been offered sweet foods for solace or comfort when they were small they may well now turn to such foods again and will rapidly put on weight. This becomes a vicious circle as they become an object for teasing and fun among their peers and a source of discomfort to themselves. They will become depressed and eat more. They are embarrassed to join their friends and play the normal games and so they take less and less exercise.

These are the girls we often meet in our Slimnastics groups. They are brought along by mothers, sisters or friends, even in a few cases by their fathers. They need sympathy and encouragement to make the best of themselves but usually they are quick and eager to take themselves in hand and with time and hard work a swan gradually emerges from the cygnet!

It is impossible to have any ideal statistics for young teenagers as they develop at such varying stages. It is, however, quite easy to detect the 'fat' from the developing. Some unhappy girls of this age have no extra fat at all but they convince themselves that they have and they become anorexic.

Anorexia Nervosa

This is a state of extreme self-maintained starvation in the presence of plenty of food and is a serious disease most common among adolescent girls but occasionally found in boys. It is not only the feminine fatness conferred by puberty which they are attempting to curb but also the biological and reproductive maturity that it heralds. As they go on slimming, menstruation ceases altogether. It is much more than just a desire to slim, it is a deep psychological wish to remain the dependent child with her family. Spontaneous recovery can occur and about 40 per cent will have recovered five years after the onset of the disease but about 5 per cent of this sad isolated group starve themselves to death. It is essential to get the right psychiatric help as soon as possible. It may well be the whole family who need help and not only the patient herself. It is very rarely indeed that we see the true anorexic in our Slimnastics groups as they go to extra-ordinary lengths to hide the fact that they are not eating. Occasionally they can be brought along by anxious mothers and then we refer them for the professional help they need.

Those girls who have been anorexic and have recovered can make wonderfully mature members of Slimnastics groups. They are very knowledgeable about foods and their values, very helpful to others, and determined never to get into that state again.

The Menopause

After their fortieth year all women can be reasonably certain that the menopause or climacteric is not so far away. The periods will gradually stop for good and it will be impossible to conceive. It is amazing to think that not so very long ago life really did come to an

end at 40 for many women who died or were dying worn out with
childbearing and disease. Although the average age of the menopause has probably not changed much since ancient times, the proportion of women reaching menopausal age has increased rapidly
with the use of reliable methods of contraception and the increase in
the overall expectation of life. As surveys have shown that less than
20 per cent of women go through the menopause without symptoms,
it is not at all surprising that there is a steady increase of interest in
the subject in the hope of extending that percentage.

The menopause is not a sudden process. It describes the gradual
changes which take place when the body of a woman stops being
capable of childbearing. First of all these changes involve the glands
of the body which produce various hormones. These in turn influence
the ovaries which eventually stop producing the tiny egg cells and
then the womb ceases to shed its lining each month so the monthly
periods stop. When the change of life begins (and it occasionally
does so in women under 40) the periods may become scanty or heavy,
frequent or infrequent. Sometimes they stop abruptly. Usually they
have ceased completely by the age of 55.

For quite a number of women the change of life takes place
gradually and comfortably but for many the hormonal changes can
create havoc with their normal heat-control, leading to hot flushes,
sweats and tingling sensations. There may be other symptoms too
which make life uncomfortable and unhappy. There are three different symptoms which can be experienced during the menopause:

1. *The autonomic symptoms* which include hot flushes, sweats, tingling sensations and gastro-intestinal disturbances. These can be
embarrassing and sometimes disturb sleep. They are probably
related to lack of oestrogen and can be reversed by hormone replacement therapy. There is no doubt about the value of this treatment
but there is still some controversy and research being done on the
subject as not all women are able to take these hormones without
undesirable side-effects. It is also not always readily available. These
symptoms can be reduced by cutting down on strong tea and coffee
and also alcohol. They can be triggered off by tension and excitement,
so taking plenty of exercise and practising relaxation is of great
benefit.

2. *The somatic symptoms* are related to changes in the mucus mem-

branes, particularly of the vagina and the urethra, and also to loss of minerals from the bones. These symptoms are also related to hormonal changes but unfortunately are less easy to reverse once established. The loss of minerals from the bones can result in the 'dowager's hump' and rounded back; also brittle bones which can easily fracture with only a minor fall. The doctor can help if the vagina becomes too dry, making intercourse uncomfortable. There is no medical reason to give up intercourse during or after the normal change of life. Some women do lose interest in sex and they should seek help from doctors who specialize in this subject. Other women, freed from the worry of pregnancy and contraception, find their sex lives are better than before. Before the age of fifty, and if your periods have stopped, use the usual contraceptive methods for complete safety.

3. *The psychological symptoms* such as anxiety, misery and irritability. These may have little or no direct connection with endocrine factors and it has been shown that the link between the menopause and severe depressive illness is probably coincidental. There is little doubt that women who have had their families, enjoy a secure and happy marital state and are adjusted to the fact that their fledglings are about to fly the nest, find they are able to deal with their menopausal symptoms with a fair amount of equanimity and a sense of humour. The same applies to women who are enjoying their work and have thought out their plans for their life ahead. It is much more difficult for those women who, needing children, have had none, or who have in other ways found life unfulfilling. They may find it very worrying to have to face the change, and dread the time when they will have no periods and the loss of what, to them, makes a woman really feminine. Some can become very depressed and disturbed. Most women probably feel passing regrets that life is going by so fast and this together with the hormone changes shows in short temper, edginess and fatigue. Doctors can help relieve these symptoms but this is a time when family and friends can be even more help. Fortunately we are today so much more aware of how our bodies work and we can talk about our feelings and problems with less inhibitions and embarrassment.

We find our Slimnastics groups can be both hilarious and helpful when discussing the problems people face during this time of life.

The groups emphasize the need for a good mental approach assisted by physical fitness. Being really fit is an essential asset in providing the energy to alleviate stress by controlling the tension.

Exercise

During the menopause this is more necessary than ever! When the natural bounce of youth has settled and children are less physically demanding, a woman is probably taking less exercise than ever before. It may be a case of a trip in the car to work, an elevator up to the office and ride down again to the car park, and a drive home perhaps to an evening in front of the television! The joints can become stiff and unused, muscles slack and posture poor. The body may feel tired, aching and aging and probably looks that way too. Exercises soon refresh the soul as well as the body. It is never too late to get the adrenalin flowing through the body again. Middle-age spread need never happen (see Fig. 27).

Look again at your diet

No longer do the insurance companies' ideal-weight charts allow extra pounds for the increasing years! There is no reason why the weight should not keep down to the ideal set for height and bone structure, but after 40 it might be much harder work and the eating pattern may need radical rethinking. With less to do and the hormonal changes going on in the body, any extra weight might be more difficult to lose. Even 2 extra teaspoonfuls of sugar (50 calories) a day more than needed will in one year add up to 18,250 calories. One pound (0·5 kg) of stored fat contains about 3,500 calories. So that in a year the body weight would increase by 5 lb (2·3 kg) and in 5 years this would add up to 2 stone (12·7 kg)! Perhaps increased alcohol consumption is doing the damage. A cool, clear appraisal of your eating pattern and its contents is needed to remain healthy enough or perhaps even live to enjoy that quarter of a century of new life ahead.

Hysterectomy

Sometimes it might be necessary to have the uterus surgically removed. If this is done before the change of life the periods will stop

Tummy and Spare Tyre (Abdomen)

Fig. 27

2 beats per picture. Practise and then put sequence together.

Starting position

1. Arms at shoulder level. Turn and touch opposite hands at one side then the other

2. Twist sideways and touch right elbow to lifted left knee

3. Twist and touch opposite hand and foot. Lift one leg straight up

4. Side bend. Join hands one side then the other

but hot flushes and other symptoms will not occur until the natural time for the menopause. If, however, it has been necessary to remove the ovaries as well then the change of life will be precipitated. In these cases doctors may well recommend hormones to make up for those usually produced by the missing ovaries. Just as after child-birth it is essential to do some pelvic exercises to strengthen up your natural girdle and put your insides back into shape as well. You will be given exercises by the physiotherapist in hospital but we give you some to do daily after you get home (see Fig. 28). There is no reason why your figure should not be as good if not better than before.

Some patients are so glad to be rid of their symptoms that they recover quickly and feel better than before, others feel a natural depression because there is no further chance of childbearing. They need a doctor's help to tide them over their reaction to the opera-tion. A hysterectomy is a major operation and it is important to realize that it will take time to recover your full strength. Follow the advice given at the hospital about gradually returning to normal life.

Maturity

Eating well for health and energy

Many older people suffer from malnutrition resulting in lack of vitamins and possibly anaemia, which can make one tired, lethargic and depressed. They may be eating badly, often because they find it difficult to buy, prepare and cook just for themselves. This may be because of loneliness, illness, unhappiness or depression. Eating should be fun for all ages and healthy eating makes for good health, longer activity and independence. This can be achieved by joining one of the local authority cookery classes, or a luncheon club, or cooking a meal regularly for a friend. During illness there will be a branch of the social service which can probably help. An emergency store should be kept for the days when it is impossible to get out. There are some ideas for easy tasty recipes for one in our cookery chapter page 103. Every day the foods in the diet must cover your basic needs for repair, resistance and energy. Our chapter on food is just as important to the older generation as it is for children, and like them it may be necessary at this stage of life to take supple-

Post-hysterectomy Static Exercises for Abdominal and Pelvic-floor Muscles

Fig. 28

Do exercises slowly – one at a time first. Try same exercises kneeling and standing. Keep breathing throughout exercises.

Starting position

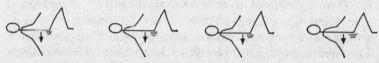

1. Contract abdominal muscles, push back into floor hard and hold. Harden buttocks. Tilt pelvis forwards

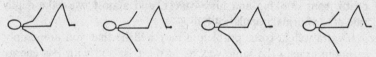

2. Harden buttocks and hold – tighten bottom hard. Contract back passage, front passage

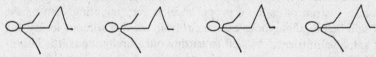

3. Grip legs and knees together really hard – let go. Pull up inside, as if to stop your waterworks

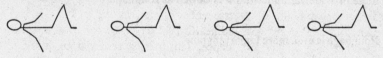

4. Tighten tummy, bottom, legs and waterworks. Hold. Now tighten abdominal muscles, buttocks, knees, pelvic-floor muscles. Pull up inside and hold again

mentary vitamins and iron. The doctor will advise you, but they can be bought very cheaply at the chemist.

Take care of your weight

Obesity is a killer and excess weight should not be ignored. Not many fat people survive into old age. It is not surprising. Several stones of excess fat strain the heart and lungs causing breathlessness, which in turn restricts activity and leads to still further deposits of fat. There is additional weight pressing on the surfaces of the hip and knee joints aggravating arthritis. Many fat people suffer from sweating and sleepiness and are unhappy about their appearance. They are also more likely to get diabetes, bronchitis, coronary thrombosis and strokes. Their expectation of life is considerably shortened. In fact the risk of death due to obesity is greater than the risk of death from smoking and lung cancer, and almost twice the death rate of the normal population!

If extra weight is the problem it may well be that you are simply eating in exactly the same way as in the past and with less energy expended to use up the food, it is being converted into fat. On the other hand, living alone, nibbling at biscuits, cakes, sweets and chocolates instead of eating a proper meal is very tempting. As we have said before, these foods can be cut from the diet without losing any valuable nutrients. As well as cutting out starchy foods it is important to cut down any excessive eating of fats. It is much better to eat foods such as potatoes, wholemeal bread, fruit and vegetables as these provide valuable vitamins as well as roughage.

Roughage is even more important now

As we have seen, roughage provided by fibres of cereals, vegetables and fruits forms useful bulk in the bowel and helps to prevent constipation. It is also helpful in the prevention of diseases of the colon and bowel. Apart from the comfort it is important to keep the bowels moving regularly. Constipation alone can create incontinence of the bladder and occasionally of the bowel too. Coarse brown bread has more roughage than white bread; coarse or medium oatmeal has more than rolled oats. Bran products added to a favourite cereal or to fruit or a milk pudding provide very useful bulk. If you have had your teeth removed or have badly fitting dentures do not avoid these foods. Chop or mince them until your false teeth have been fitted or adjusted.

Water

This can help with constipation too and it also helps prevent bladder infections. Eight cups of fluid are necessary every day but this should be increased during hot weather or during illness if there is fever or vomiting. Do not restrict drinking because you are afraid of having to 'get up in the night,' an old-fashioned 'potty' is a great asset!

Exercises in the bath

On page 216 (see Fig. 29) are some gentle exercises designed to do in a warm bath. Not only is the bath a support but the therapeutic effects of exercise in warm water are many. In the first place the warmth helps to relieve any pain and induces relaxation, and as the pain in the joints or muscles is relieved the body can move more easily with both greater comfort and increased range and this increases the blood supply to the skin, improving its condition and any poor circulation in the extremities such as the fingers or toes. As the warm blood reaches the underlying muscles and their temperature rises they contract more easily and more strongly but tire less quickly.

You may feel generally rather limp after you have been exercising in a hot bath. This is nothing to worry about but it is wise to keep warm and rest for a while to allow the heart, respiratory and metabolic rates as well as the distribution of the blood to return to normal.

Sex is good for the heart!

The wise men of India and China used to think that regular sexual activity was the key to eternal youth. Certainly sex is very good exercise for the heart and lungs and can be enjoyed into a ripe old age. Sexual desire continues throughout life for both men and women though potency or the ability to perform the act may fall off gradually. Even if the complete act becomes difficult or impossible

Exercises in the Bath

Fig. 29

Do exercises slowly. Gently stretch the joints. Use soft mat in bath to kneel on.

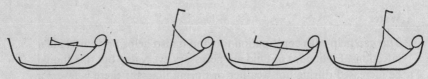

1. *Strengthening abdominal muscles, mobilizing knees, hips, ankles, feet. Loosening hamstrings*

Hold position as far as you can. Then do foot exercises – turn foot up, down and circle

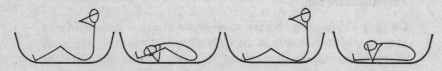

2. *Stretching hamstrings and mobilizing back and shoulders*

Hands behind head, elbows forwards, legs bent or straight legs apart. Reach down elbows between legs

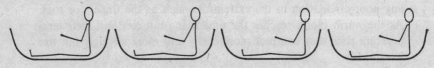

3. *Strengthening the legs, arms, hands and fingers*

Press both legs towards outsides of bath and hold. Press both arms towards outsides of bath and hold. Hand exercises in the water – clench, stretch – fingers apart – together

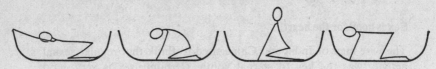

4. *Ankles, knees, hips, shoulders, back, head and wrists*

Slowly go from one position to the other

both partners with understanding can continue to derive great satisfaction, pleasure and happiness from close sexual intimacies. The benefits of a relationship with the opposite sex in mutual companionship, comfort, happiness and love are enormous.

Keep moving to keep living

'Immobility is a short cut to growing older quicker', said the splash headline in a magazine. It is quite true. Regular exercise has far reaching effects and it is never too late to start. Studies have been carried out among elderly people who have for years been leading an inactive life. The group who began to include exercises in their daily routine not only became fitter but actually seemed younger in every way. They had increased the strength and mobility of their limbs and joints; exercise also stimulated their adrenal glands which had helped them regain some of their youth and give them confidence. More important to their health, their blood chemistry had improved, the blood-fat levels and the blood-clotting levels had dropped. Their blood pressure had improved and their pulse rate when resting was lower and returned more rapidly after exercise. There is no doubt that exercise is good for you but discuss with your doctor which form of exercise is the best for you personally.

Most people do not wear out, they rust into immobility! Start by walking everywhere you can. If walking is difficult take to the bicycle – it takes the weight off the feet but does wonders for the joints (see Figs. 30 and 31). If this does not appeal, take to the water. Swimming is excellent exercise at any age. Many authorities run special classes for adults and there are usually special rates for pensioners.

Join an exercise class. Our Slimnastics groups for the elderly are full to bursting point and our other Slimnastics groups have many pensioners in them too. The exercises are nearly all supported by the use of chairs, the floor or a partner so that no harm can come to backs, joints or muscles which are not as strong as they were. These groups deal with the weight problem too and afford plenty of opportunity for discussions and talk which can be of great benefit to those whose usual audience is the cat or the radio.

Easy Exercises for Stiff Joints

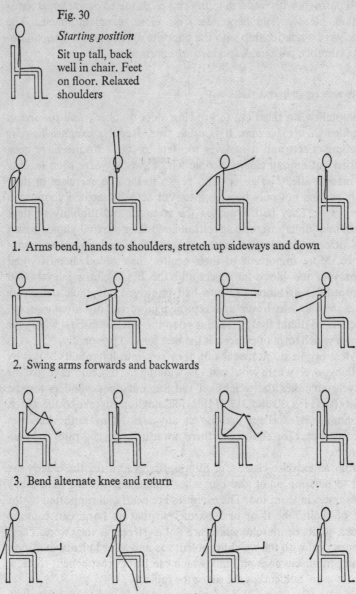

Fig. 30

Starting position

Sit up tall, back well in chair. Feet on floor. Relaxed shoulders

1. Arms bend, hands to shoulders, stretch up sideways and down

2. Swing arms forwards and backwards

3. Bend alternate knee and return

4. **One** leg stretch, sideways, centre and down

Shoulder-joint Exercises

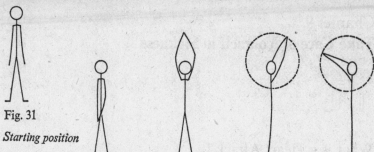

Fig. 31

Starting position

1. Fingers intertwined – raise both arms above head – circling above head

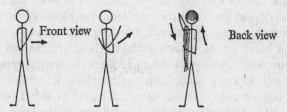

Front view   Back view

2. Touch left hand on right shoulder. Push a little further, with right hand on left elbow. Repeat. (Towel over one shoulder as if drying after bath)

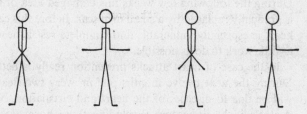

3. Keep elbows into sides, move forearm across and out

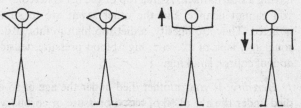

4. Press elbows back as hard as you can

Chapter 9
Take Care of Yourself in Sickness

What is a Heart Attack?

The heart is a muscular pump sending the blood round the body with oxygen and food for the tissues. The heart muscle cannot get the oxygen and food for itself from the blood circulating inside its own chambers, and so two arteries called coronary arteries supply the heart on its outside surface. These arteries can become very narrowed as you grow older and the walls become roughened. If the blood clots at a particularly narrow place, stopping the flow, this is called a coronary thrombosis (heart attack) – derived from thrombus (clot) in a coronary artery. A small area of the heart muscle is now deprived of blood carrying fresh oxygen and food. This causes severe pain across the chest, often extending to the neck and arms and the area may be large enough to cause the patient to collapse. During the following few weeks this damaged area of the heart wall is gradually replaced by a small firm scar. Before this can happen the heart is especially vulnerable and complete rest is needed to give it as little work to do as possible.

In the case of heart attacks prevention really is better than cure. During the next twelve months one in every two deaths in Britain will be due to diseases of the heart and circulation. Many of these deaths will be premature. Excluding those born with damaged or deformed hearts there are eight ways of increasing your risk of having a heart attack. At the top of the list is heredity which is a fact you cannot change, but the other seven are to some extent self-inflicted. They are obesity, a diet too high in fats, a diet too low in roughage, lack of exercise, high blood pressure, tension from stress and, of course, smoking.

1. Heredity: If your mother died under the age of 55 or your father died under the age of 60 of blood pressure or coronary heart disease you must take extra care not to inflict the other seven burdens on your body. On the other hand if either or preferably both parents lived to a ripe old age of 80 or more you will have a built-in survival kit.

2. Obesity: The death rates go up about 13 per cent for each 10 per cent of excess weight. Being 20 per cent overweight makes you 25 per cent more likely to have a heart attack. For most of us there is no medical reason why we should be overweight. It is almost always due to drinking or eating too much. A large fat body gives severe muscular strain to the heart, since it has to flush blood through all that fat and carry nutrients around the body in increasingly restricted capillaries.

3. A diet too high in fats: The fat layers on our bodies, which are made up from the fat, protein and carbohydrate of our diets, are quite easily burned off for energy and produce few waste products, since the main result is carbon dioxide and water which we exhale. The difficulties involved in over-eating fat lie in the complex cholesterol molecule always found in conjunction with animal fats.

This tends to make cholesterol a very frightening word, but it is in fact a natural substance produced by the liver. The blood transports cholesterol from the liver, where it is made, to the other parts of the body where it is needed. The other way our bodies can obtain cholesterol is directly from foods which already contain it, such as eggs, brains, liver and hard fats.

Young babies need cholesterol for their brains to develop properly and adults need it for the formation of such vital substances as sex hormones. However, some people produce too much cholesterol and this is when the trouble starts. The body does not have a simple way of burning it up and it can become stockpiled. Before long the blood can become saturated with it and it can fall out of solution and form deposits which can be very difficult to shift. This blockage or clot in the artery can pose a serious threat to the heart.

Most doctors and nutritionists recommend that the amount of fat in the diet is reduced to lower blood-cholesterol levels rather than by cutting out very nutritious foods like eggs. It is the hard fats like butter, lard and hard margarine which provide little more than one nutrient – fat – and these are therefore much less valuable items of diet. A person does not have to be overweight to have a high cholesterol level but cutting down fats in the diet does have the added advantage to those who are overweight in that it is so very high in calories.

Obviously here we are thinking of prevention and not cure. If a man or woman has recently had a heart attack or is known to be at a very high risk they may be advised to take more drastic dietary measures. They must listen and take heed to the advice of their doctor or dietician.

4. A diet too low in roughage: There has recently been a medical report published in Great Britain which demonstrates a link between dietary fibre and the prevention of heart attacks. Among a survey of men over a period of 20 years, it was those whose diet contained a significantly high roughage content who had the least heart attacks. A diet containing lots of fruits, vegetables and grains will increase the bulk of the stool and shorten the time it spends in the colon. Furthermore, high-fibre diets tend to fill you up before you have consumed more calories than your body really needs and again this helps to prevent obesity.

5. Lack of exercise: Regular physical activity protects against heart disease. The body deteriorates if you do not use it. It is the sedentary people who have a higher heart-attack rate than the active ones. Isometric exercise, which is physical activity involving sustained muscle contractions such as weight-lifting and 'press-ups', can be dangerous for people with heart disease or high blood pressure because of the resulting strain on the heart. It is dynamic exercise – physical activity in which muscles contract and shorten in a rhythmic manner, such as jogging, running, walking and swimming – which is best for improving the functions of the lungs, heart and blood circulation.

The long-term health hazards of not exercising are more serious than the short-term risks associated with fitness schemes but it would be prudent to start any exercise programme gradually at first. Those who are over 35 and under 50 and have not done any exercise since leaving school should consult their doctor if they are at all worried about their health. Those over 50 should make sure to seek medical advice before starting on any fitness scheme. Under 35 and under-exercised they should start slowly but without delay!

A considerable amount of exercise can be taken unobtrusively by walking or cycling to work, avoiding escalators and lifts in favour of walking up the stairs, joining a Slimnastics group, a businessman's gym and in gradually working up to playing squash. Many men and women find the ideal solution in jogging (see how to get started on this in Chapter 6, page 158).

6. *High blood pressure*: Taking heed of the five points above will possibly be the answer to lowering your blood pressure. On the other hand hypertension may need further medical help and any advice from your doctor should be taken seriously. It might be advisable for men over 40 years of age to have a complete medical check-up every three years.

7. *Tension from stress*: As you will have seen in Part III, Relaxation for Fitness, tension in the muscles affects the mind and vice-versa. Physical health goes a long way to giving you the strength to deal with the stresses of life. Exercises can also give positive relaxation to the muscles and this will be transmitted to the mind. Many a man coming back from a jog or drying after a swim finds it difficult to recall just what it was that was worrying him so much! He can now see things in perspective.

It is easy to think that alcohol is an aid to relaxation. If the tension is all in your head the alcohol may relax you and as alcohol is a sedative it will certainly make the tense person feel better. However, it has been shown that the drinks have no effect on the tension in the muscles. Exercise first and then perhaps a drink is a better answer.

8. *Smoking*: The safest smoker is the non-smoker. However, if you stop heavy cigarette smoking at, say, the age of 50, you will carry the same risk as a life-long non-smoker by the time you are 60! So it is worth making the supreme effort to stop. Any patient who has had a heart attack should stop cigarette smoking immediately and most of them do so without much difficulty. Pipe tobacco, cigars and whiffs carry a much reduced risk which basically amounts to not inhaling.

Recovery and convalescence

Immediate post-coronary advice must come from your doctor or the hospital as every case can be so very different. But as you get stronger there is no doubt that you will be advised to put into operation the points above which apply to you. With thought, determination and some effort you may soon feel better than you have for a long while.

Early Detection of Cancer

Examine your breasts

Try to make the examination of your breasts a monthly habit; possibly immediately following a period or on the first day of the month if you have had the menopause. If there is something wrong with the breast, it is far better to find it by monthly self-examination than to wait to discover it by chance. Even cysts and non-malignant tumours and growths are more easily dealt with while they are small. Breast cancer can be treated very successfully when it is diagnosed in the early stages. The success rate is now approaching 80 per cent in early cases.

Undress to the waist and examine your breasts. These are the warning signs you are looking for:

Unusual difference in size or shape of the breasts.
Alterations in the position of either nipple.
Retraction (turning in) of either nipple.
Puckering (dimple) of the skin.
Unusual rash on the breast or nipple.
Unusual prominence of the veins over either breast.
Unusual discrete lump or nodule in any part of either breast.

If you have any doubts, visit your doctor, local Family Planning Clinic, or Well-Woman Clinic and they will help you. Encourage your friends to do the same.

The cytotest

The cytotest is a simple early detection test for cancer at the entrance to the womb. It is wise to have regular smear tests done before, during and after the menopause. The cytotest picks up many small things that are not cancer at all so do not worry if your doctor asks you to come back for further tests. He may be able to treat these problems easily and save you trouble later on. If, however, the tests show that cancer might develop, a small operation to remove a tiny area of the cervix might be necessary. Having this test does not mean that you will never get this type of cancer, but if you have the test regularly it does mean that this particular form of cancer can be discovered at a very early stage and never be given a chance to develop. Remember that the cytotest could save your life and every woman over the age of 35 should make an appointment to have one regularly from her own doctor or the local clinic.

Cancer in men

Unfortunately, it is not possible for men to detect cancer by self-examination.

Recurring Ailments

Many of us seem to acquire at least one recurring ailment which seems sent to try us! Some of these are irritations which seem too minor to merit seeking medical help but they are nevertheless annoying and sometimes worrying too. Other conditions respond to medical attention, only to keep reappearing at intervals with seemingly no prospect of a permanent relief. We are asked for basic information about these ailments so often by members of our groups that we thought it worthwhile compiling a list of those which came up most frequently. If your particular interest is not in this list it may well be mentioned elsewhere in this book. However, we fully expect to have to add to this list in subsequent editions.

Acne: This results from the overactivity of the sebaceous glands. This leads to the blocking of the ducts, which in time leads to blackheads, red papules and pustules. This can cause scarring. Dirt does not cause acne but it can make it worse. On the whole diet, with the exception of chocolate, makes little difference. It is a tiresome, stubborn and demoralizing problem. It mainly occurs from puberty to the age of 25.

Unfortunately the worse it gets, the more germs thrive and the worse the skin condition becomes. The first priority is hygiene. Use the specially prepared antiseptic soap which you can buy from the chemist; keep to your own face towel and change it frequently;

change your pillow-case nightly to avoid the spread of infection; keep your hair clean (and of course brushes and combs); avoid touching the affected area, but if a pimple is rubbed or scratched then you should wash your hands immediately. You can buy antiseptic soothing creams especially for this condition. Put it on with cotton wool and throw this away after use. Astringents may also be useful to help dry up excess oil in the skin.

Alcohol: Like smoking, alcohol has its dangers. An occasional drink is both sociable and pleasurable, it is habitual heavy drinking which is bad for you. Exercise speeds up the combustion and disposal of alcohol; and oxygen helps the circulation and tissues to deal with it. It is much better not to assault the body with too much alcohol, but if you do ever suffer from a hangover you will need plenty of fluid as the chemical processes by which the body breaks down and utilizes the alcohol cause dehydration. So a brisk walk in the open air and drinking plenty of WATER should do the trick! Alcoholism is an illness and needs professional help. There are societies which have been formed to advise and support both the alcoholic and the relatives.

Allergies: An allergy is a reaction of the blood to the presence of a foreign substance, usually a protein. Unfortunately the reaction of the blood is to produce histaminic acid which is both useless and harmful. It can affect the sufferer in many different ways and in so many different parts of the body. Some of the most common effects can be asthma, catarrh, hay fever, migraine, skin complaints. The most common precipitants are a wide and varied list from animals, pollens, foods (such as beetroot, strawberries and chocolate) and alcohol, to house dust and mites, any drug, nickel or chlorine, and even the sun.

Allergies can be hereditary but this is not always so. Avoiding the cause is the best method of treatment but this may not be easy and is often impossible. Much research into the subject is resulting in better and safer anti-histamines. If you have recurring or prolonged 'colds', skin complaints or migraine headaches it is wise to think back and see if you can find a common factor. You might be able to identify and thus avoid the substance altogether, or, if this is impossible, have a course of desensitizing injections or take an antihistamine. In this way you may decrease or even rid yourself of the effects completely. There is a good book on food allergies, *It's Not All In The Mind*, by Richard MacKarness (Pan, 1976).

Alopecia: This is a strange but quite common condition when small bald patches appear on the scalp, even on the heads of quite young children. It is believed to be of nervous origin and often follows some nervous strain or disturbance. It nearly always recovers spontaneously and the hair soon grows normally again. It is not infectious.

Athlete's Foot: This is a fungus disease which can not only be painful but unpleasant to your family or colleagues. The early symptoms of this complaint are excessive peeling of the skin and tenderness between and under the toes. If immediate action is taken with proprietary ointments the trouble may be eliminated in a very short time. Those who suffer excessive perspiration of the feet are most prone to this disease and should take the advice on hygiene of the feet, page 178. If the trouble persists, seek the advice of a doctor or a chiropodist.

Boils: A boil is an infection in a tiny gland in the skin. The germ responsible, the staphylococcus, enters through the duct from the gland and is particularly likely to do so when the area is damaged by friction. This is why boils occur most frequently on the buttocks, the back of the neck and under the arms. They do not necessarily indicate any defect in general health. Heat applied with poultices and hot fomentations brings the boil to a head and hastens recovery. Never squeeze the boil or the infection is likely to spread. A course of penicillin is sometimes necessary.

Bunions: A bunion is a painful red lump, which develops at the side of the base of the big toe, when the toe has become angled towards the other toes. A sac of fluid forms under the skin causing the prominent lump over the bone. At first it acts as a protection but with increasing pressure it becomes reddened and inflamed.

A bunion develops because the toes have been continually bunched up together in tight socks or shoes. Once it has formed, the only curative treatment is an operation to straighten the offending joint. However, you can help yourself in the early stages by wearing shoes that are wide enough and putting a small pad of wool between the big toe and the next one so that it does not get bent any further.

Car-sickness: There is no one single cause for this distressing complaint, so there are correspondingly numerous 'cures'. Travel pills can be a great help but they vary greatly. Read the instructions and follow them carefully. They are powerful drugs – do not mix them with alcohol. They should never be taken by the driver as they might make him drowsy. The driver is usually immune to car-sickness but it is a point to remember for those drivers who take tablets to quell a queasy stomach on a cross-channel ferry. They may well be a danger to themselves and others as they drive off the boat at their destination. Travelling with children is an art – but in avoiding sickness, plenty of distractions and no book-reading is generally a good rule and plan your journey during their sleep periods whenever possible.

Chilblains: Chilblains are red or bluish-red itching swellings which appear in cold, especially in cold and damp, weather. They are mostly seen on fingers and toes, but also on the outer ear and on the lower part of the calf of the leg. They are most common in children and in persons whose general health is below the average. For general treatment and prevention, improve the circulation by exercise and make sure you have adequate vitamin D in your diet.

Colds: The average person has three to four colds every year. Most colds clear up spontaneously and it is only the complications such as sinusitis, bronchitis or pneumonia which need attention. There are so many cold viruses that immunity to one does not protect you from others. Although much research has been done into prevention and cures, only little progress has been made. Vitamin C is said to help but there is not much evidence as yet to prove this. It does help to clear the nasal passages and prevent any blockages of the sinuses if you inhale regularly with boiling salt-water or Friar's Balsam. Some colds make you feel quite low and it is wise to include extra vitamins in your diet and give yourself time to build up strength again.

Constipation: It is not necessary to have a bowel motion every day. Constipation is caused by the faeces being hard – not simply because the bowels have not moved for 48 hours. It is important to eat a diet with plenty of roughage – wholemeal bread, wholemeal cereals, bran, fruit and vegetables – and drink at least 4 to 5 pints (2 litres) of liquid a day. Never delay going to the lavatory. Regular exercise will help too by strengthening the abdominal muscles which will help the bowel movement. If the constipation does not respond to increased roughage in the diet or mild laxatives, it should be treated by the family doctor.

Cystitis: This is an inflammation of the bladder. It is caused by an infection with any one of a number of different germs and can be associated with other conditions of the bladder. It is more common in women but does occur in the older man. Usually cystitis can be cured in a few days with drugs but sometimes the germ proves resistant and with some people this condition recurs with distressing frequency. In women cystitis can sometimes follow intercourse and a self-cure in this case is to empty the bladder very soon after intercourse. After going to the lavatory take care to wipe yourself from front to back to avoid infection spreading. There are some helpful books on the subject, particularly those by Angela Kilmartin, who started the Cystitis Society, the address of which can be found in a public library or local Citizen's Advice Bureau.

Dandruff: Dandruff is sometimes due to a disorder of the sebaceous glands of the scalp. It is difficult to treat and it is wise to seek expert advice before trying out the different preparations which are available. There is no evidence that dandruff is catching but we all have germs present on our scalps and these tend to multiply in people suffering from this condition.

Dyspepsia: People who suffer from frequent bouts of indigestion should make sure that they eat regular meals and never go for long periods without food. Little and often is the golden rule. Try having 5 small meals a day. Take plenty of time over your meals too. Avoid all fried and spicy food and also rich sauces. If it persists seek medical advice.

Gout: Sufferers from gout have an alteration in the chemical processes of the body. This tendency to produce too much uric acid is normally inherited from one or the other parent or grandparent. The uric acid may form crystals which appear in, and around, joints and sometimes elsewhere such as on the ear. One of the aims of treatment is to prevent the accumulation of these crystals and to get rid of them if they have formed. With modern drugs this is now perfectly possible, even in the more severe cases. Too much alcohol is not the cause of gout but it can 'trigger off' an attack, so can too much food, too much worry or fatigue. Injury, even a small one, can trigger off an acute attack of gout. Always be on the look-out for the early signs of an acute attack if you suffer from this complaint. The earlier you start treatment the better, for at first gout will do no permanent damage to the joint but if it is left it can start off a condition of chronic arthritis.

Headaches: A headache is a symptom, not an illness in itself. It can occur for many reasons; for example, illness, accident, arthritis of the neck, high blood pressure, tension, eye strain, sinusitis or migraine. It can also of course be the result of a hangover!

An intense headache of sudden onset in an otherwise healthy person who is not known to suffer from migraine merits an urgent visit to the doctor. A mild headache of short duration which does not recur can safely be ignored. A mild headache of short duration which keeps recurring should be investigated. You need to search for the cause. Make an appointment with the doctor.

Once you have established that your headache is not the symptom of something more serious but perhaps the result of tension, pre-menstrual syndrome or even a stuffy room, a short sleep, a rest, change of occupation, or walk in the fresh air may ease the pain.

Heartburn: This is a feeling of heat at the lower end of the breast-bone, usually occurring an hour or more after a meal. It has nothing to do with the heart, but results from an acid reflux from the stomach into the gullet. It is particularly apt to follow the taking of fatty or fried foods. It can be quickly relieved by the taking of milk or an alkali such as bicarbonate of soda in water. To prevent heartburn avoid all indigestible foods, avoid stooping, and if necessary use an extra pillow at night. If it persists seek medical advice.

Herpes: These cold sores are due to a virus infection. The lip is the commonest site of the infection and after the first attack the virus may lie dormant in the tissues under the skin and a new attack may be triggered off by a cold or similar infection or even by sunlight. Surgical spirit applied with cottonwool will help.

Lice: Unfortunately, lice have reached almost epidemic propor-tions. They live in the head, waist and pubic regions of man. The eggs of lice which stick on to the hairs are called nits. These cause discomfort and irritation and certain types of lice may transmit serious diseases. Do not hesitate to go to your doctor or health clinic for advice and help. Excellent treatment is available. Take especial care of personal hygiene for the whole family as lice can spread quickly from one person to the next.

Migraine: In migraine the blood vessels of the brain are especially sensitive and liable to attacks of abnormal dilation. These attacks are often preceded by a period of vaso-constriction (spasm of blood vessels) which gives warning of the approaching headache. The severe headache is usually only on one side of the head, is associated with vomiting, blurred vision and sometimes temporary paralysis, particularly on one side. Migraine is often triggered off by tension or allergies. Severe and frequent migraine should be treated by the doctor and he may refer you to a special clinic if necessary.

Moles: Moles are merely small patches of pigment concentrated in the skin and are perfectly harmless. If you notice any difference in the size, shape or colour of your mole consult your doctor as they can occasionally give trouble.

Phobias: A phobia is a condition in which the amount of fear experienced is excessive in relation to the cause. These are much more common than one thinks and not easy to deal with. Some people are lucky enough to find that they get this condition only in special circumstances such as claustrophobia (fear of closed spaces like lifts) to vertigo (fear of heights). Others are not so fortunate and if the fear becomes so unreasonable that it seriously disrupts your life you will have to seek a cure. The fears can be of many things varying from enclosed spaces, wide-open places, heights, flying, spiders or thunderstorms. If you feel it is getting out of hand, consult your doctor and he may well refer you for further help. There are specialized societies which help those suffering from common phobias. The addresses are available from libraries and Citizens' Advice Bureaux.

Piles or Haemorrhoids: These are dilated veins which may be internal or external. External piles are felt as little lumps which itch, and which are apt to become hard and inflamed. Internal piles occur inside the bowel, but after evacuation they may prolapse and be visible externally as soft swellings which can usually be pushed back with a finger. Internal piles are apt to bleed and when inflamed they cause a discharge which may be blood-stained. They also cause a desire to evacuate the bowel, and the congestion caused by the attempts to do so aggravates the condition. Treatment is aimed at first correcting the constipation which is almost always a forerunner. Ask your doctor's advice about a laxative and pile ointment and adjust your diet to include more roughage. If the piles continue to cause distress by pain or itching, especially bleeding, ask for medical advice. They may need surgical treatment by injection, removal or stretching the anus. Piles which occur during pregnancy can be the result of pressure and these will probably soon recover after the birth.

Psoriasis: Psoriasis is often a familiar condition in which there is a persistent or recurrent scaly skin rash over different parts of the body. It can also affect the joints or nails. It is not infectious or contagious in any way, rarely occurs on exposed areas and tends to clear up for long periods by itself. There is as yet no really effective remedy for this condition but many new methods of treatment are being tried out, so consult your doctor and get his advice. In severe cases psoriasis can be very distressing because of its appearance. There is a Psoriasis Society which is very helpful.

Sebaceous cysts: These develop in the tiny skin glands which secrete a lubricating material. If the outlet from one of these glands becomes blocked the gland swells up into a cyst full of this lubricating matter and it may grow even to the size of an egg. They are quite harmless but can be removed under local anaesthetic if necessary.

Snoring: Anything which causes mouth breathing as opposed to breathing through the nose is liable to result in snoring. Children with enlarged adenoids may snore, so may people with persistent nasal catarrh, sinusitis and nasal polyps. Dealing with these conditions may cure the snoring. However, there are others who snore without any real reason. The only resort for those who have to sleep with them may be earplugs!

Teeth grinding: Many people grind their teeth from time to time during sleep, but they do not always know that they do it. There is no reason to fear that it will harm the teeth; it may do them good. Teeth clenched through tension may well impact a nerve and that is very painful indeed and you must seek the cause of the tension.

Threadworms: These are white thread-like worms and easily seen on a stool. There is no need to feel ashamed to consult your doctor about this very common condition. It is by no means normally limited to children; adults are very frequent sufferers. Treatment, with tablets or medicine is simple, rapid and effective. It is usually necessary to treat the whole family as 'recurrence' is probably a reinfection. Until the condition has been cured you must pay strict attention to the ordinary rules of hygiene – handwashing after using the lavatory and before handling food. The eggs of the threadworms tend to lie under the nails, so nail-biters are most at risk!

Varicose veins: A varicose vein is an abnormally dilated, tortuous vein. It is caused by the weakening of the walls of the vein as a result of obesity, constipation, long periods of standing or pregnancy. There is most probably a hereditary factor. Walk as much as possible, avoid standing for long periods and wear support tights or socks. Sit with your feet up and legs firmly supported. If necessary raise the end legs of your bed. In mild and moderate cases injections may cure the veins. In more severe cases an operation may be necessary.

Warts: Warts are caused by a virus, they are ugly but they do no harm. No one has yet established why they come or why they suddenly disappear. Orthodox medicinal remedies often do not seem to have any effect and warts are sometimes claimed to be cured by 'magic' or 'granny's patent cure'. This is most likely due to the fact that most warts spontaneously disappear anyway – but you never know!

Chapter 10
Taking Care of Others in Emergency

Accidents do happen, at work, at play, travelling, and in particular to the young and the elderly. Many of the effects of these accidents can be minimized if prompt action is taken. We often want to help but do not know how or what to do.

The very best advice we can give you is to go and undertake a course on first aid. The Red Cross runs many and they are well publicized. It is very difficult to learn heart massage and artificial respiration without a practical demonstration and regular practice. You should also own a first-class first aid manual which will give full details of dealing with any situation. We can only deal here with various remedies in brief but we hope our notes will be of use or serve as reminders should the necessity unfortunately arise.

Remember: Do not delay learning about this very practical way in which you can be of help to others – to wait might prove fatal.

Be Prepared – The Emergency First-aid Cupboard in the Home

The cupboard, or small case or box, should be readily accessible to adults but locked or impossible to open by children. It should not be kept in a damp atmosphere (a bathroom is not a suitable place). Bottles and containers should be clearly labelled and should have tight-fitting, preferably screw caps. Dressings should be in small packs so that any unused material is unlikely to be left over inadequately wrapped. Replace any items that have been used at the earliest opportunity.

This first-aid kit should contain:

Soluble aspirin, 25 tablets
Paracetamol, 25 tablets

Anti-histamine cream, 1 tube
Calamine lotion, 180 mls
Methylated Spirit, 120 mls
Disinfectant, 1 small bottle
Roller bandages, $2 \times 1''$, $2''$, $3''$
Conforming bandage, $1 \times 3''$
Triangular bandages, 4
Prepared sterile dressings, $1 \times$ small, medium, large
Assorted adhesive dressings, 12
Adhesive strip dressing
Gauze, $3 \times \frac{1}{2}$ yard packets
Cottonwool, $3 \times \frac{1}{2}$ oz packets
Adhesive plaster, $1''$ wide roll
Paper tissues, 2 small packets
Safety pins, mixed sizes
Scissors, 1 pair, blunt-ended
Forceps or tweezers
Clinical thermometer
One small bowl or plastic kidney dish
Torch with spare bulb and battery
Bisodol, Alka-seltzer or your own favourite tummy settler.

The first-aid kit which you should keep in your car should contain a smaller quantity of the items named above but plus some money for emergency phone calls and also a packet of car sickness pills. It is also useful to keep a plastic sheet in the car for any casualty to lie on and a rug to keep them warm. You should also keep a pencil and notebook handy.

Help – Emergency!

As we have said, it seems to us of prime importance that everyone should take a first-aid course. However, first aid does not take the place of professional help. By your telephone should be a note in clear writing. It should show the telephone numbers of your doctor, your local casualty hospital and your local police station. It should also have boldly printed your name, address and telephone number – in a state of panic anyone can forget even where they are, and remember the casualty might be You! It is no good all the information being stored in your head if you are lying unconscious and need the help.

We give below a few basic tips to help you in the event of an emergency. If you are in any doubt do not hesitate to call for medical attention. Prompt action can save lives. *Never* give anything by mouth if the casualty is likely to need medical care. A full stomach delays giving an anaesthetic and this means more pain. With minor injuries that need hospital attention it is sometimes quicker to use your own or a neighbour's car rather than call for an ambulance. Never panic! Whenever any emergency occurs the casualty needs to be calmed down and treated in a reassuring manner.

Bleeding (severe): Press firmly directly over the wound for 10 minutes. Keep the casualty at rest and elevate the wounded part if possible, unless you suspect a fracture – a broken bone should not be moved. Dress the wound and immobilize it. If necessary treat for *Shock* (see below) and send for help.

Burns and Scalds: Cool immediately by immersing the injured area in tap cold water until the pain has gone, usually at least 10 minutes. Cover with a clean dry dressing once the burn has cooled and if necessary treat for *Shock* and seek medical aid.

Drowning: Give *Artificial Respiration* and *Heart Compression (Massage)* if necessary. Seek urgent help.

Electric Shock: Switch off the supply, pull out plug or tear the cable free (be careful not to touch any conducting material yourself). Give *Emergency Resuscitation (Artificial Respiration)* and *Heart Compression (Massage)* and send urgently for medical aid.

Emergency Resuscitation (Artificial Respiration): See Fig. 32 on page 240. If the casualty has stopped breathing, do not hesitate, act promptly and methodically and you might well save a life.
(a) Very quickly remove any obvious obstruction in the mouth or any constriction round the neck or chest.
(b) Lay the casualty on his back, press his head backwards with one hand until his nose is pointing nearly directly upwards, push his chin forwards so that it juts out. This will raise his tongue from the back of his throat and he may start to breathe.
(c) If not, pinch the nostrils shut with the fingers of one hand.
(d) Take a deep breath, open your mouth, seal your lips round the casualty's open mouth.

(e) Blow air firmly and gently into the mouth and so into the lungs. Do not blow harder than is necessary to keep the chest moving. (For small children and babies seal your lips round both mouth and nose. With a child blow more gently, for a baby small puffs are sufficient.)

(f) Remove your mouth, turn your head and watch the chest fall.

(g) Repeat about 4 times and watch to see if natural breathing has begun. If not continue at a steady deliberate rate about 12 times per minute, watching the rise of the chest as guarantee that air is going into the lungs and blowing in again as soon as the chest has fallen. Seek help urgently.

Epilepsy: This condition may occur at any age, but usually first appears in young people. Persons with epilepsy are liable to recurrent attacks, which may be of two types, minor and major; the latter may also be due to an addict taking an overdose of a stimulant drug.

Minor epilepsy (petit mal) – The condition may resemble a fainting attack and should be treated as such. The individual becomes pale with eyes fixed and staring and is not conscious of his surroundings. He may then resume his previous activity as though nothing has happened. Watch should be kept for the presence of post-epileptic automatism (as described below).

Major epilepsy (grand mal) – This is a true epileptic fit. The person sometimes has a premonition that he is going to have a fit. He may experience a sense of strangeness accompanied by a headache, irritability, restlessness or a feeling of lethargy – the 'dreamy state'. These sensations, if they occur, are quite brief.

The fit consists of 4 stages:

1. The person suddenly loses consciousness and falls to the ground sometimes with a cry.
2. He remains rigid for a few seconds, during which time his face and neck become congested and cyanosed.
3. Convulsions, consisting of alternate contraction and relaxation of groups of muscles, begin. There is noisy breathing through a clenched jaw. Froth sometimes comes from the mouth and will be blood-stained if the tongue is bitten. He may lose control of the bladder and bowel and pass urine and motions involuntarily (incontinence).
4. The casualty then reaches the stage in which his muscles become relaxed.

On regaining consciousness, he has loss of memory for recent events and may be dazed and confused and need a little while to gather himself together. He may act in a strange way and wander about without realizing what he is doing (post-epileptic automatism); this condition varies in duration. He may then feel exhausted and fall into a deep sleep.

First aid – The aim is to prevent the casualty, who has no control of himself, from receiving any injury and to keep his airway clear.

1. Restrain the casualty only as far as is necessary. Forcible restraint of an epileptic may cause injury. Guide, but do not restrict, his movements.
2. Protect him from danger – fire, water, any object against which he might injure himself.
3. As opportunity arises, remove any false teeth and put a knotted handkerchief or similar firm 'bite-on' between his jaws, as far back as possible, to prevent his tongue being bitten. Do not prise open his mouth.
4. Wipe away any froth from the mouth.
5. Apply the general treatment of *Unconsciousness* as far as is required.
6. Keep careful watch for a possible recurrence, and do not leave him until you are satisfied that he is fully aware of his surroundings.
7. Advise him to see his doctor or, if necessary, send him or take him to hospital.

Fainting: Lay the casualty back and raise the legs about 18 in (46 cm) off the floor.

Foreign Objects: In the Eyes – limit your assistance to a very gentle wash out of the eyes with tepid water and send the casualty to an out-patient department. Eyes are delicate organs and should be left to the experts.

In the Nose – do not try to poke the object out. Tell the casualty to breathe through the mouth and seek medical aid.

In the Ears – particularly in children. Do not attempt to remove the object. Take the casualty to an out-patient department.

Fractures or Dislocations: Immobilize not only the fracture site but also up to and beyond the joints on either side. You can immobilize by securing to a part of the casualty's body, e.g. leg to leg.

Keep the casualty at rest and if necessary treat for *Shock* (see below) and send for or seek medical help.

Head Injury: Treat the casualty for *Shock* and seek medical attention even if there is no outward sign of injury. There may be a delayed reaction.

Heart Attack: Place the casualty in a comfortable position – semi-recumbent (head and shoulders raised) or supported in a sitting position. Loosen clothing at the neck, chest and waist. Be quietly reassuring but send for medical aid *urgently*. See *Heart Compression* (*Massage*).

Heart Compression (*Massage*): If after four successful movements of the chest by artificial respiration, the casualty's colour remains deathly blue-grey, the pulse cannot be felt and the pupils are widely dilated, you can be certain that the heart has stopped. Immediately try to restart its action.

(*a*) Strike the breastbone sharply with the hand once or twice (with babies tap sharply with two fingers). This may start the beat.

(*b*) If this does not succeed, place the casualty on his back on a firm surface (preferably the floor). Elevate legs.

(*c*) Kneel by the casualty. Put the 'heel' of one hand on the lower hand – keeping your palms and fingers off the chest (see Fig. 32 on page 240).

(*d*) Press just above the lowest inch of the breastbone, press down firmly but evenly by rocking forward on your straight arms.

For adults: 60 times a minute.

For children: 80 times a minute (using the heel of one hand).

For babies: 100 times a minute (using the pressure of two fingers only).

Success is judged by the colour improving, the pupils contracting and the pulse returning.

Muscle Cramps: These may be relieved by stretching the cramped muscles in the opposite direction to the cramp and by applying warmth or rest. If the cramp follows excessive heat and sweating give the casualty a drink of water containing half a teaspoonful of salt to the pint (that is $\frac{1}{4}$ teaspoonful to the tumbler).

Muscle Strains: Warmth and rest!

Fig. 32

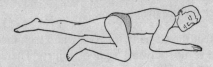

1. The recovery position for the unconscious or resting casualty

2. *Artificial Respiration*

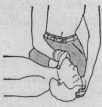

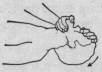

3. *a* Lie the casualty on his back. .

b Press the head backwards with one hand until the nose is pointing nearly directly upwards, push the chin forwards so that it juts out. Pinch the nostrils shut.

c Take a deep breath, open your mouth, seal your lips round the casualty's open mouth. Blow air firmly and gently.

d Remove your mouth, turn your head and watch the chest fall.

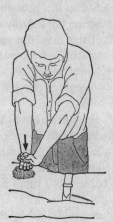

4. *Heart Compression* – put the heel of one hand on the lower hand keeping your palms and fingers off the chest.

Nose Bleed: Sit the casualty by an open window with his head bent slightly forward and loosen any tight clothing. Tell the casualty to pinch the whole soft (lower) part of his nose firmly for 10 minutes and warn him not to blow his nose for some hours. If the bleeding continues seek medical help. The casualty should breathe through his mouth and spit out blood into a bowl instead of swallowing it.

Poisoning: Gas and exhaust fumes – provide fresh air and give artificial respiration if breathing has stopped.

Non-corrosive poisons such as drugs – make casualty vomit by tickling the back of his throat. If this fails give drink of water containing 2 heaped tablespoons of salt per ½ pint (284 ml).

Corrosive poisons such as disinfectants, cleaning fluids, petrol – give the casualty water or milk to dilute corrosive. Do not make him vomit as this may make burns worse. Yellow, grey, or white burns around the mouth betray corrosive poisons.

In all cases send an urgent message for ambulance or doctor. Explain what is the suspected poison and ask for advice about anything else to be done in the meantime. Preserve any remaining tablets, medicines, containers or vomit for the doctor to examine.

Shock: This dangerous state of physical collapse develops after heavy bleeding, severe injuries, burns or fractures. The casualty becomes very pale and cold, with a moist skin, fast weak pulse and breathing. After you have treated any obvious injury, move the casualty as little as possible. Lay him down putting something soft under his head. Turn his head to one side in case he vomits. Raise his legs above head level (unless they are fractured). Loosen any tight clothing round the neck, chest or waist. Keep him warm with blankets, rugs or coats under as well as over the body (never use a hot water bottle). Send urgently for medical help but stay with the casualty and keep him calm and reassured.

Sprains, Bruises and Swellings: A cold compress held with a crêpe bandage is useful. Rest the injury and obtain medical attention if in any doubt of the severity of the damage.

Suffocation: First remove the obstruction (for instance the plastic bag over the child's head, the cord round the neck, etc.). For sudden choking give several hard thumps between the shoulder blades (a child may be held firmly upside-down while this is done). Make sure air passages are clear – keep the head bent backwards and the lower jaw pressed forward. Start *Emergency Resuscitation* if necessary and treat for *Shock*.

Unconsciousness: If the breathing has stopped start *Emergency Resuscitation* at once. If there is bleeding control it; but otherwise put the casualty in the recovery position:
Lying on one side.
The leg and arm of that side behind him.
The other arm and leg bent in front, with the knee and elbow at about a right angle.
The head tilted slightly backwards and the face turned slightly towards the ground.
Clear the mouth of any obstruction (blood, froth, vomit). Remove false teeth and loosen clothing at the neck, chest and waist. Examine and give any further treatment required. Place blankets or coats above and below the casualty and get medical aid. *Never* give any food or fluids or leave the casualty alone.

Part V
Slimnastics for You

Having read the book so far, you will have a pretty good
idea of the whys, the wherefores, the theory and the practice
of exercise, nutrition, relaxation and your life cycle. We hope
that you are by now convinced that a passive interest, even
if accompanied by excellent intentions, will do you no good
at all! It is positive action that is needed – but most of us
find that while the spirit is willing the flesh is very weak!
Prevention may sound better than cure, but unless there is
some urgent medical reason or we have already experienced
pain and discomfort, we easily slide into the decision to do
something about it – tomorrow, another day, or at least
sometime soon!

We started Slimnastics back in 1964 based on the
principle that achieving good health and fitness through
exercise, sensible eating and relaxation of body and mind
was very difficult on one's own, whereas the Slimnastics
group encouraged the achievement of these aims, prompted
discussions and exchange of ideas and assisted members of
the groups not only to help themselves but support each
other. It succeeded quite beyond our wildest dreams. Not
only are there many small home groups doing Slimnastics,
we now train professional Slimnastics leaders who already
have qualifications in movement, teaching, physiotherapy or
dietetics and they run Slimnastics groups in adult colleges,
further education, schools, health clinics, clubs and offices
not only in the U.K. but several other countries. We never
lack group members, in fact most of our groups have waiting
lists.

Chapter 11
The Slimnastics Ten-week Fitness Plan

Everyone has at least one part of their body which they wish to improve. In this chapter we give you a guide to a ten-week course that each person can adapt to suit their needs. There are also the Exercises for the Body, which will mobilize joints and strengthen muscles all over the body (see Figs. 55–73). These can be done once a week alone or in a group. If you are reasonably fit and require something more challenging to improve your stamina and strength, the Fitness Circuit (see Figs. 51–4) is for you. You can go from stage to stage at your own pace. There is a chart (see Appendix 1) on which to mark your progress.

One word of warning. We feel that it is very difficult to assess one's own degree of physical fitness. Of course you are obviously not at your best if you are overweight, have arthritic hips, have just had flu or are on medication of any kind. On the other hand, we meet people who tell us they are very fit, play tennis every day and eat well but who even so feel very stiff after a course of exercises and are found to have a diet high in fat and low in roughage! Take no chances; if you feel it is at all necessary, check with your medical practitioner. He is more than likely to be delighted that you are taking positive steps to improve your health and decrease his workload but he knows your body better than you do – so be guided by him.

In any event, we feel that everyone will benefit from starting slowly and gradually increasing the activity they put upon themselves. We have set plenty of challenges along the route, but it is better to arrive there safely than fall by the wayside.

246 Slimnastics for You

Introducing the Ten-week Fitness Plan

Time plan:

1. Daily exercises for 7 minutes.
2. Daily relaxation for 5–10 minutes.
3. Once a week an exercise session of 40 minutes.

Exercise plan (every day for 5 days in the week):

1. Two minutes spent (morning or evening) doing the Stretching exercises (see Figs. 33–4).
2. Five minutes doing exercises of your own choice from the Fitness Course of Exercises (see Figs. 35–50). Start at Stage 1 and progress week by week at your own rate.
3. Five–ten minutes on relaxation: 2–5 minutes on the exercises for relaxation.
   2–5 minutes on total relaxation.
   As you get more proficient you can spend more time on the complete relaxation.

Once a week:

1. Weigh at the same time each week on the same scales in the same clothes.
2. Do a 40–60-minute exercise session *either* with a Slimnastics group (see Figs. 55–73 – Exercises for the Body),
   or   in a gymnasium or exercise club,
   or   work through the Fitness Circuit (see Figs. 51–4),
   or   do some form of sport.

Ideas to help you through the ten-week plan

Week 1: Exercises and relaxation. Weigh and measure yourself. Fill in the Personal Statistics Chart (see Appendix 4). Fill in the Diet Sheet (see Appendix 7) with complete honesty!

Week 2: Weigh yourself. Exercises and relaxation. Take a good look at your completed Diet Sheet. Read Chapter 3, Food for Health, and underline your mistakes. Create a healthy eating pattern which suits you and stick to it.

Week 3: Weigh yourself. Exercises and relaxation. Readjust your eating, and plan if necessary. Read Chapter 4, Cooking and Eating for Fitness, and try out some of the ideas.

Week 4: Weigh yourself. Exercises and relaxation. Read Part III, Relaxation for Fitness, and become especially aware this week of tension in your muscles; learn to tense and relax.

Week 5: Weigh and measure yourself. Fill in the Personal Statistics Chart (see Appendix 4). Exercises and relaxation. Be aware of your 'stress signals'; how do you blow your top? Think of positive ways to help yourself.

Week 6: Weigh yourself. Exercises and relaxation. Read Chapter 8, Take Care of Yourself and Others Throughout Life, in particular those sections which apply to you or members of your family. Take appropriate action.

Week 7: Weigh yourself. Exercises and relaxation. Read Chapter 9, Take Care of Yourself in Sickness, and Chapter 10, Taking Care of Others in Emergency. How well equipped is your first-aid kit? Have you done a first-aid course? If not – it is time you enrolled!

Week 8: Weigh yourself. Exercises and relaxation. Take a look at your outward appearance. How good is your skin? Is your hair in good condition? Do your clothes look as good as you feel? Do your shoes have a comfortable fit?

Week 9: Weigh yourself. Exercises and relaxation. Consider the activities mentioned in Chapter 1, Exercise and the Body. Choose an activity mentioned under the part of your body which most needs exercises and one which appeals to you and go and try it!

Week 10: Weigh and measure yourself. Complete the Personal Statistics Chart. Exercises and relaxation. Plan to celebrate with one of our special menus in Chapter 4. If you have a group, you can all bring one of your favourite slimming dishes and have a celebration lunch or supper. It's a good opportunity to swop recipes.

Chapter 12
Course of Exercises for Groups

This is not as difficult to get going as you might think:
1. Start with a nucleus of people – not too many, perhaps only three or four. You will soon gain more members if you want to and the number of people is limited by the space available.
2. You will need a small cleared area such as the living-room floor, office or club room. Each person needs enough space to be able to lie down comfortably with arms outstretched. The room should be warm and airy, the floor clean and comfortable – wooden blocks or carpets are very good, floor tiles or concrete can be very cold.
3. You will need one chair per person, bathroom scales, tape-measures and comfortable clothing. (There is no need to wear leotard and tights, tracksuit or shorts. A T-shirt and stretch trousers are equally as good. Jeans are unsuitable as they inhibit the movements of your legs and trunk.)
4. Each member of the group will need a copy of this book! They have got to discover about nutrition, exercise and relaxation for themselves.
5. You will need some kind of sustenance after the exercise session; such as low-calorie cool drinks, tea or coffee.
6. You will find it much more enjoyable to do the exercises with music, in which case you will need a tape-recorder or record player. Each exercise can be done to the beat of four though it is not necessary to keep in time.

The Slimnastics Class

Measuring

At the first meeting measure each other and record the results on the Personal Statistics Chart (see Appendix 4). The moment of truth has arrived! Do not chicken out. Even if you do not need to lose weight, the exercises will improve your shape and when you record the results at the end of the ten weeks you will be very pleased. Do remember that muscle weighs heavier than fat so that some of you who are of under or average weight may even gain on the scales as the weeks progress. However, you will look better for it! Remember when measuring to check that the tape-measure is around the correct part of the anatomy and not twisted or pulled too tight.

Weighing

Although you measure only at the beginning, middle and end of the ten weeks, everyone weighs every week. Weigh each other, not only to prevent cheating but also because it is impossible to get an accurate reading from above. No bathroom scales are completely accurate, especially if they are kept in the bathroom, cloakroom or kitchen, as the steam corrodes them and they rust. Nor should they be used on a carpet as this upsets the balance. You should make it a rule always to use the same set of scales in the same place at the same time each week and you will get quite an accurate assessment of losses and gains. Discourage any comparison with any other scales as this may well be disconcerting.

Decide on your weight aim

This all depends on how much you have got to lose. You can find this out by looking up the Ideal-weight Chart (see Appendix 5). If you have a lot to lose, unless otherwise medically advised, 1 stone (6·4 kg) in the ten-week term is an achievable aim. For those of you with not so much to lose, 1–2 lb (0·5–0·9 kg) a week weight-loss will keep you looking and feeling good. The last 7 lb (3 kg) are the hardest to lose and do require some effort. However, it is worth the struggle, as the last pounds are the ones which make all the difference. Try to end up with a few pounds in hand. This will allow for the holiday binge!

Setting the scene

Clear as much of the furniture as possible and make sure the room is warm but well ventilated.

If the group includes young mothers with babies and toddlers, we find that it is better to have enough space to keep them in the room with us (at least you know what they are up to!) and each mother is responsible for her own child. Toys should be kept to the minimum and be suitable – wooden hammers and jolly little animals on wheels with bells can play havoc with your nerves! You will find that many of the children learn to join in and thoroughly enjoy their exercise times.

Exercises for the Slimnastics group (see Figs. 55–73)

In the first week do the exercise course for 30 minutes, and in the following weeks gradually increase the time to 40–45 minutes for the session. Either one of the group can direct all the exercises or you can take a page each in turn. TAKE YOUR TIME AND DO NOT RUSH! Take it easy. Do the exercises slowly but well. You can gradually increase the pace. If you want to make the sessions slightly longer or more strenuous, include a stage from the Fitness Course of Exercises (see Figs. 35–50), or try the Fitness Circuit (see Figs. 51–4) as you become fitter.

Relaxation

After the exercises, make sure everyone is warm enough – put on sweaters or use a rug each. Do the Neuromuscular Relaxation exercises (see pages 155–7) for 5 minutes. Take it in turns to talk through the exercises. Gradually you will learn to do it by memory.

Refreshments

Lay a tray ready for refreshments before the group meets. Then there is no delay and those who have to get away promptly can do so. This is the time to discuss the Diet Sheets and the points to be considered in the Ten-week plan.

The Ten-week plan

Follow the Ten-week plan together (see pages 246–7) as a group and do the daily exercises and relaxation on your own as well. When you have finished the ten-week course have a short break – you will soon find that you will want (or perhaps need as well!) to start again. We find that most terms have natural breaks such as Christmas, Easter and summer holidays. These happen to be the times of maximum self-indulgence too!

Fig. 33   *Daily Stretching Exercises*

Waking up in the morning. Daily stretching and mobilizing.
Do slowly and continuously – feel stretched then relaxed.

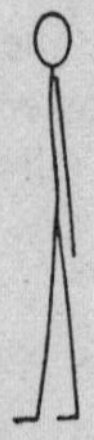

Starting position

Stand tall, relax
shoulders, tail in,
tummy in. Take two
deep breaths – in
through nose and
out through mouth

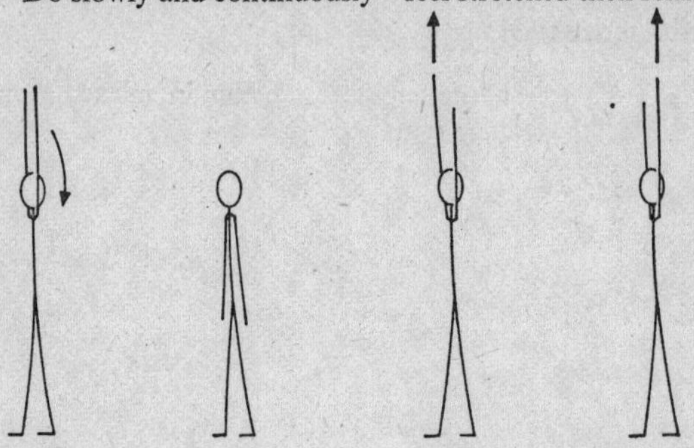

Arms circling slowly

Reach for ceiling
with an alternate arm

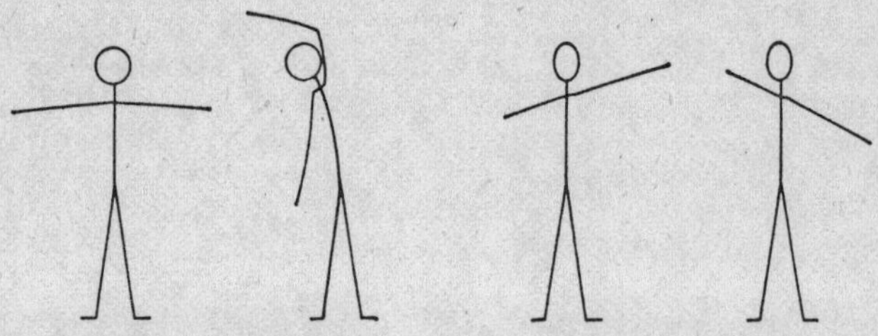

Bend alternate side
and return slowly

Twist alternate side –
look backwards

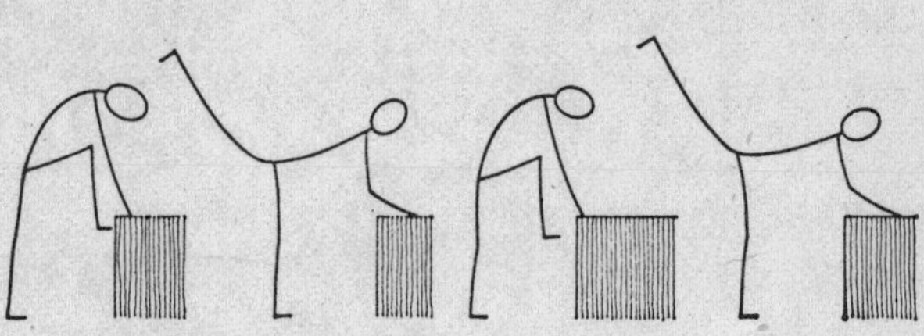

Slowly bend – stretch alternate leg

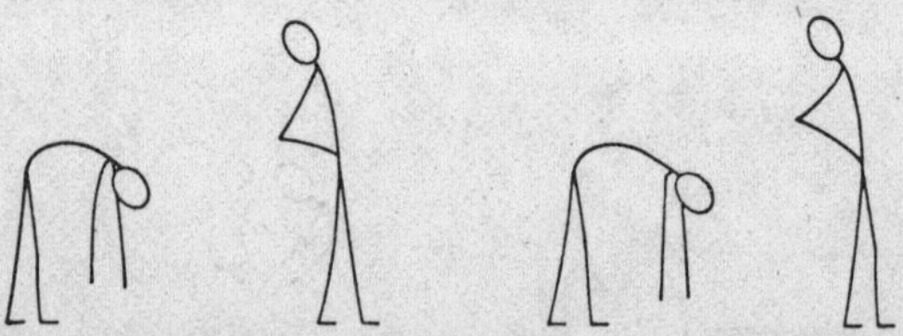

Slowly reach towards the floor then arch backwards, hands on
hips

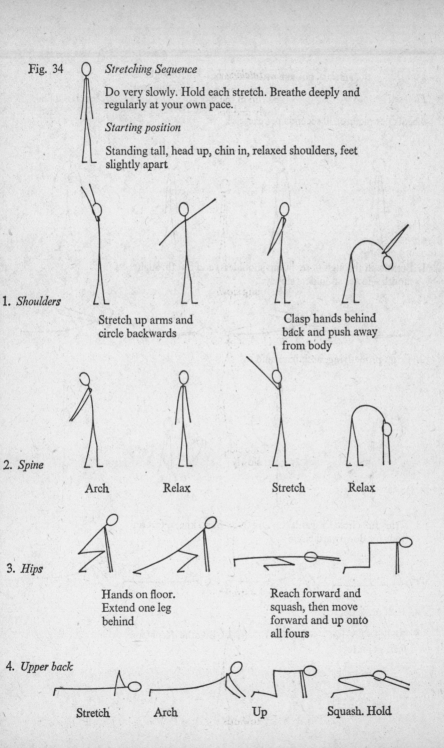

Fig. 34 *Stretching Sequence*

Do very slowly. Hold each stretch. Breathe deeply and regularly at your own pace.

Starting position

Standing tall, head up, chin in, relaxed shoulders, feet slightly apart

1. *Shoulders*

Stretch up arms and circle backwards

Clasp hands behind back and push away from body

2. *Spine*

Arch   Relax   Stretch   Relax

3. *Hips*

Hands on floor. Extend one leg behind

Reach forward and squash, then move forward and up onto all fours

4. *Upper back*

Stretch   Arch   Up   Squash. Hold

Fig. 35   FITNESS COURSE OF EXERCISES   10 exercises
(5 minutes)

Fitness 1

4 beats per picture, 30 seconds per exercise.

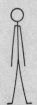 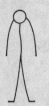 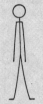

1. Breathe in through nose, hump shoulders, and out through mouth – lower shoulders slowly

   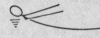

2. From prone-lying, arch back and lower

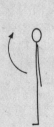 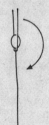 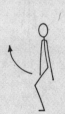 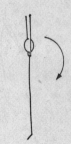

3. Arms full circle forwards, up and over. Bend knees, feet on floor for downward circle

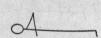 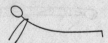 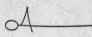

4. Half press up.

5. Walking on spot – swinging arms freely. Breathe deeply, use feet, point toes

Fig. 36

Fitness 1

4 beats per picture, 30 seconds per exercise.

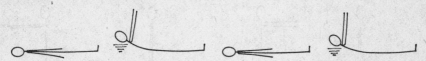

6. From lying on back, lift shoulders off floor

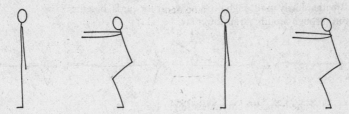

7. Keep heels on floor, knees together. Bend knees and
   straighten

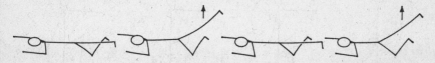

8. From lying on side, lift top leg up and down

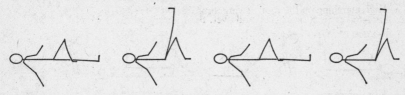

9. From lying on back, lift one straight leg up and down

10. Lying on back, relaxed, eyes closed

Fig. 37

Fitness 2

4 beats per picture, 30 seconds per exercise.

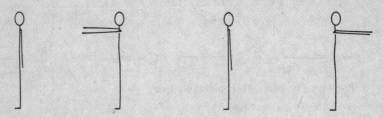

1. Breathe slowly in through nose, arms lift forwards, breathe
   out through mouth. Arms lower etc.

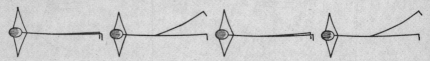

2. From prone-lying, lift alternate straight leg

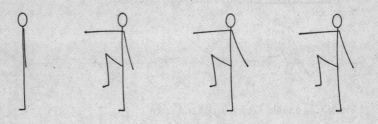

3. High marching on the spot – swing arms freely

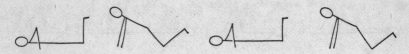

4. Knee press ups

5. Walking round room, good posture. (Heel, little toe, big toe.)
   Breathe deeply

Fig. 38

Fitness 2

4 beats per picture, 30 seconds per exercise.

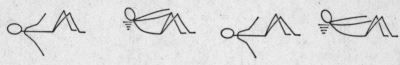

6. Touch right hand to left knee

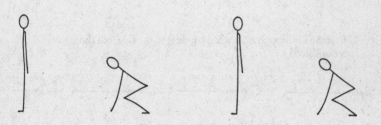

7. Keep back straight, hands on floor – bend and straighten

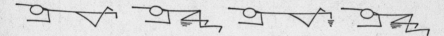

8. From side-lying, bend and stretch top leg

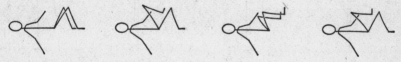

9. From crook-lying, marching. Change legs in mid-air

10. Lying on back relaxed – eyes closed

Fig. 39

10 exercises
(5 minutes)

Fitness 3

4 beats per picture, 30 seconds per exercise.

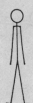 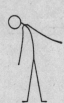 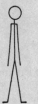 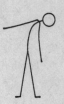

1. Breathe in through nose when bending to the side, out through mouth slowly

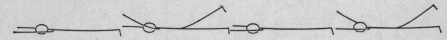

2. From prone-lying, lift opposite arm and leg

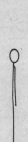 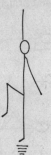 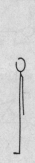 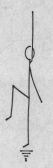

3. Leaping into air, lift alternate arm and leg

4. Hips lower and lift

5. Walking fast on the spot

Fig. 40

Fitness 3

4 beats per picture, 30 seconds per exercise.

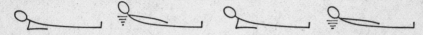

6. Touch knee caps, from elbow support

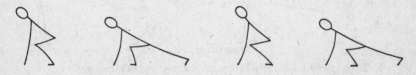

7. Stretch alternate leg behind

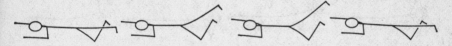

8. From side-lying, hold top leg as high as possible for 8 beats

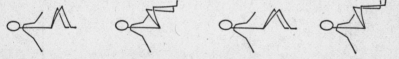

9. From crook-lying, bend knees to chest and return

10. Lying on back, relaxed, eyes closed

Fig. 41

10 exercises
(5 minutes)

Fitness 4

4 beats per picture, 30 seconds per exercise.

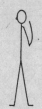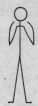

1. Twist and breathe slowly in through the nose and out through mouth when you return

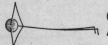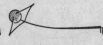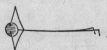

2. From prone-lying, arch back. hands behind head

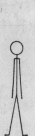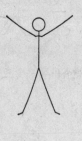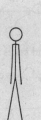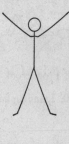

3. Star jump out and in

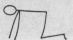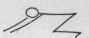

4. Reach forwards and backwards

5. Walking and jogging alternately

Fig. 42

Fitness 4

4 beats per picture, 30 seconds per exercise.

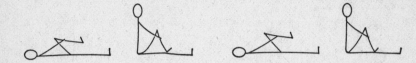

6. Change legs – sit up holding knee and return

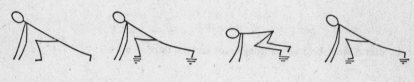

7. Jump and change legs in mid-air

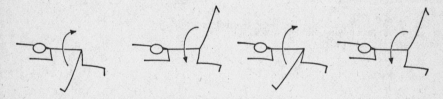

8. From side-lying, lift top leg over and back in semi-circle

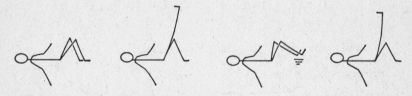

9. From crook-lying, straighten alternate legs

10. Lying on back, relaxed, eyes closed for one minute

Fig. 43

10 exercises
(5 minutes)

Fitness 5

4 beats per picture, 30 seconds per exercise.

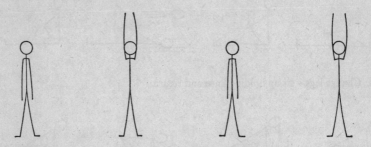

1. Stretch arms, breathe in through nose and out through mouth

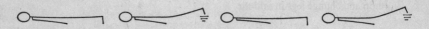

2. From prone-lying, tighten buttocks, lift legs

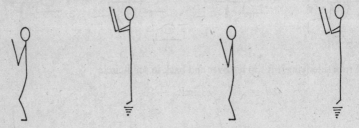

3. Use arms to give height to jump. Jumping on the spot

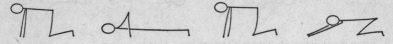

4. Straighten forwards and squash backwards

5. Jogging on spot for one minute

Fig. 44

Fitness 5

4 beats per picture, 30 seconds per exercise.

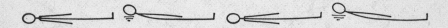

6. From lying on your back, lift head and shoulders, touch knee caps

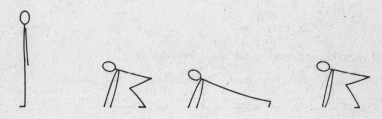

7. Jump legs behind, and stand up

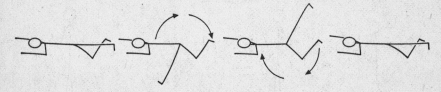

8. From side-lying, move top leg full circle

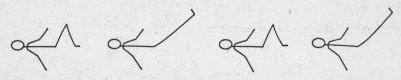

9. From crook-lying, straighten legs and return

10. Lying on back, relax, eyes closed

Fig. 45

10 exercises
(5 minutes)

Fitness 6

4 beats per picture, 30 seconds per exercise.

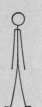 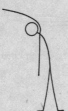 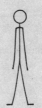 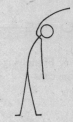

1. Breathe out through mouth and in through nose

2. From prone-lying, lift alternate bent legs, then both

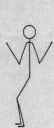 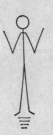 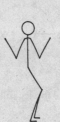 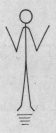

3. Jump, twisting hips before landing

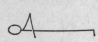 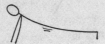 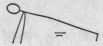

4. Three-quarter press ups. Lift shoulders, then hips, then return similarly

5. Jogging slowly and running on spot alternately, for one minute

Fig. 46

Fitness 6

4 beats per picture, 30 seconds per exercise.

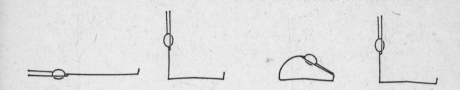

6. Swing arms up and over – chest on knees

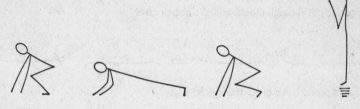

7. Jump legs out and in, and up

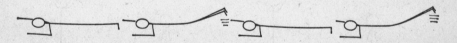

8. Side-lying, lift legs off floor and hold

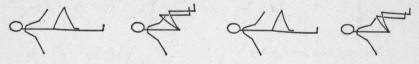

9. Cycling, legs off floor

10. Lying on your back, relaxed for one minute

Fig. 47

10 exercises
(5 minutes)

Fitness 7

4 beats per picture, 30 seconds per exercise.

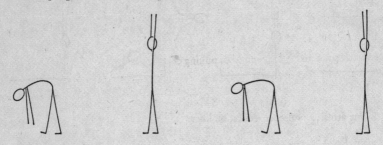

1. Breathe out through mouth and in through nose

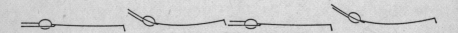

2. From prone-lying, arms and legs off floor

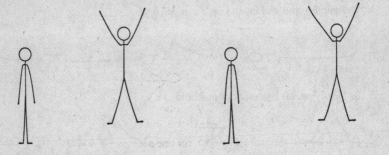

3. Star jump, land feet together

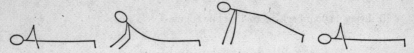

4. Up in two halves, down body straight

5. Jogging and running fast alternately for one minute

Fig. 48

Fitness 7

4 beats per picture, 30 seconds per exercise.

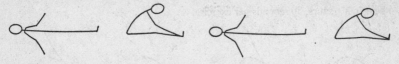

6. Hold ankles and gently bend elbows, pulling chest towards floor

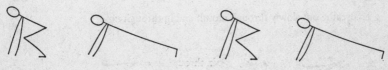

7. Jump feet away and towards hands

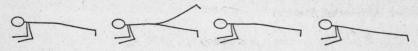

8. Front-lying, elbow support, lift hips off floor, lift one leg and return

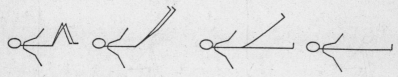

9. From crook-lying, follow stick men

10. Lying on back, relaxed, eyes closed, for one minute

Fig. 49

10 exercises
(5 minutes)   *Fitness 8*

4 beats per picture, 30 seconds per exercise.

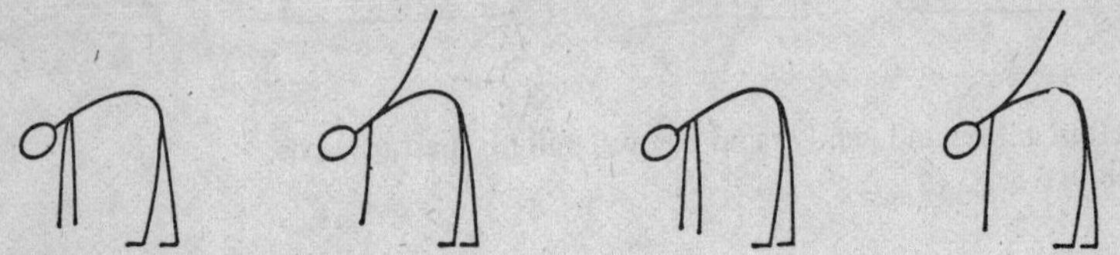

1. Breathe out slowly through mouth and in through nose

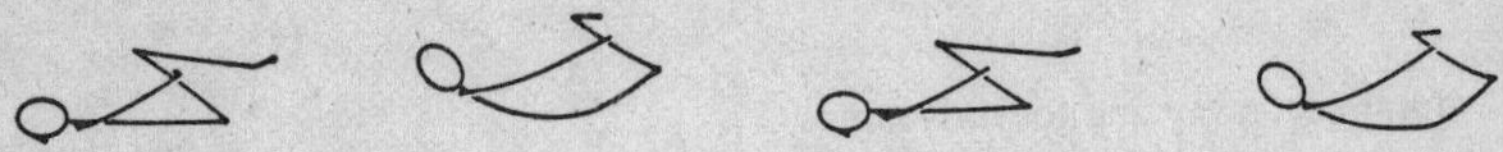

2. Arch back, hold ankles

 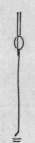 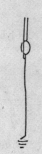

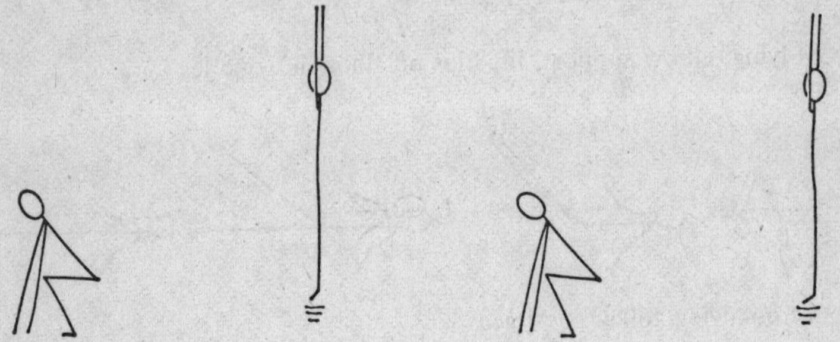

3. Squat jumps

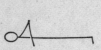 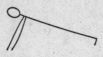 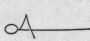 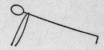

4. Press ups – straight back

5. Jogging and high-knee raising alternately for one minute

Fig. 50

Fitness 8

4 beats per picture, 30 seconds per exercise.

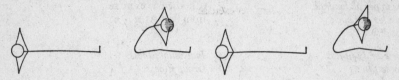

6. Hands behind head on neck

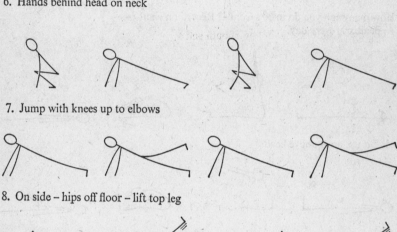

7. Jump with knees up to elbows

8. On side – hips off floor – lift top leg

9. Change legs, keep straight

10. Lying on back, relaxed, eyes closed, for one minute

Fig. 51

Fitness Circuit –
Part A

For upper abdominal
muscles and back
mobility

(Choose one exercise
from Part A)

For Family fitness
Home fitness
Holiday fitness

Individual fitness
Group fitness

How many can you do in 30 seconds? Record on chart (see
Appendix 1) every day.

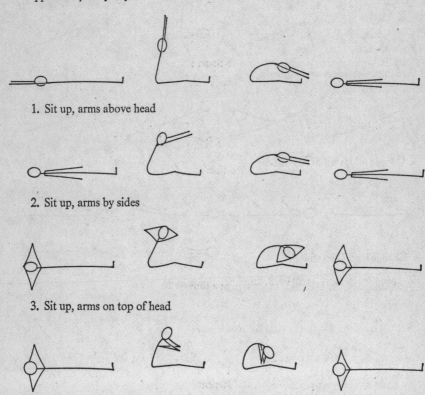

1. Sit up, arms above head

2. Sit up, arms by sides

3. Sit up, arms on top of head

4. Sit up, arms behind neck

Fig. 52

Fitness Circuit – Part B

For abdominal muscles   (Choose one exercise
and hip mobility   from Part B)

For Family   *Individual*
Home   *Group*
Holiday

How many can you do in 30 seconds? Record on chart (see
Appendix 1) every day.

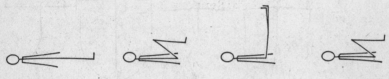

1. Bend legs, stretch, bend, straighten to floor. Repeat

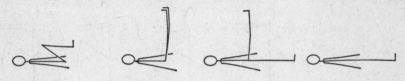

2. Bend legs, stretch, lower one leg at a time to floor. Repeat

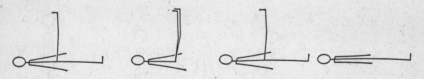

3. One leg lift, the other lift, lower one at a time to the floor.
   Repeat

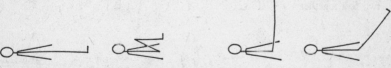

4. Bend legs, stretch and lower to 45°. Repeat

Fig. 53

Fitness Circuit – Part C

For heart, lungs, *endurance*	(Choose one exercise from Part C)	How many can you do in 30 seconds? Record on chart (see Appendix 1) every day.
For Family *Home* *Holiday*	*Individual* *Group*	

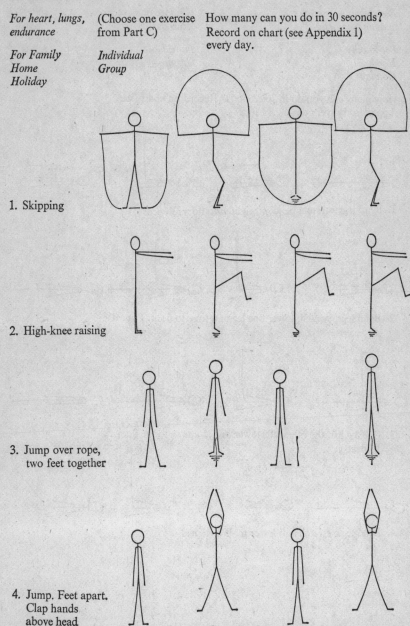

1. Skipping

2. High-knee raising

3. Jump over rope, two feet together

4. Jump. Feet apart. Clap hands above head

Fig. 54

Fitness Circuit – Part D

*For back strength –
upper and lower back*

(Choose one exercise
from Part D)

*For Family
Home
Holiday*

Individual
Group

How many can you do in 30 seconds? Record on chart (see
Appendix 1) every day.

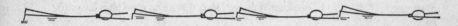

1. With feet and thighs just off ground – lift alternate legs, as in
   legs for front crawl swimming

2. Lift thighs and shoulders off floor and return

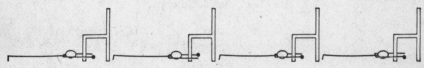

3. Make figure of eight with weight round chair leg

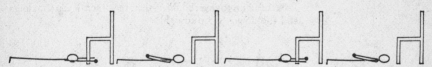

4. Pass weight round one chair leg, then behind back

Head and Neck Exercises

Fig. 55

Head and Neck Exercises

To relieve tension and strengthen neck. Do movements slowly, with no jerking. Follow sequences to music, 4 beats per picture.

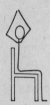

Starting position

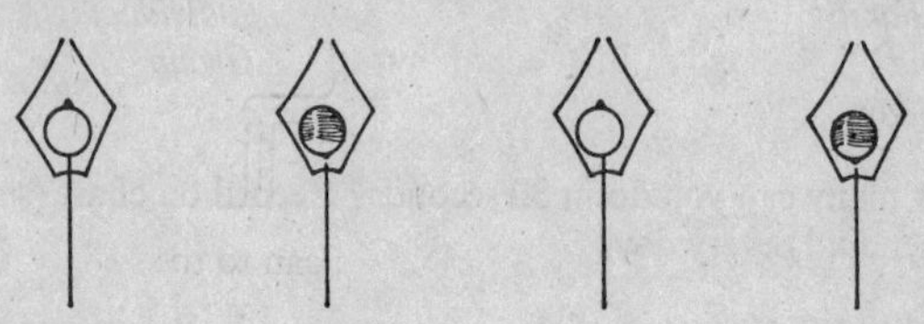

1. Look up at fingers, look down and press chin into chest

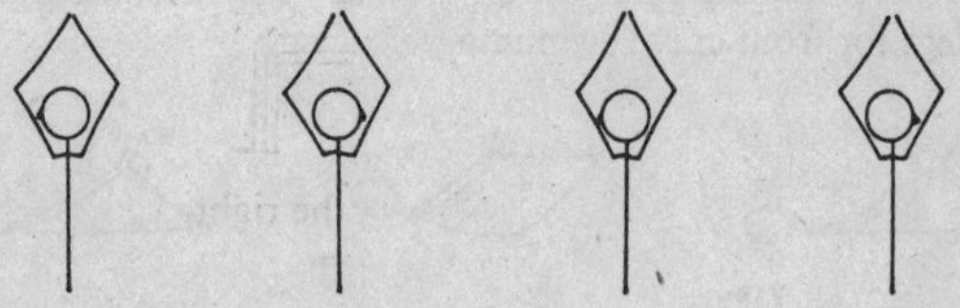

Sit tall, hips well back and into chair, hands above head, elbows back, relax shoulders. See sitting posture. Breathe naturally

2. Look at right elbow, then left, keep elbows well back, hands above head, shoulders down

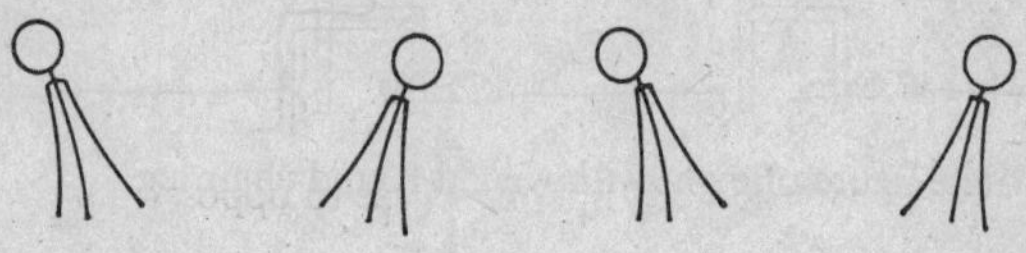

3. Press head on to one shoulder, then the other. Keep shoulders still and down. Sit up straight

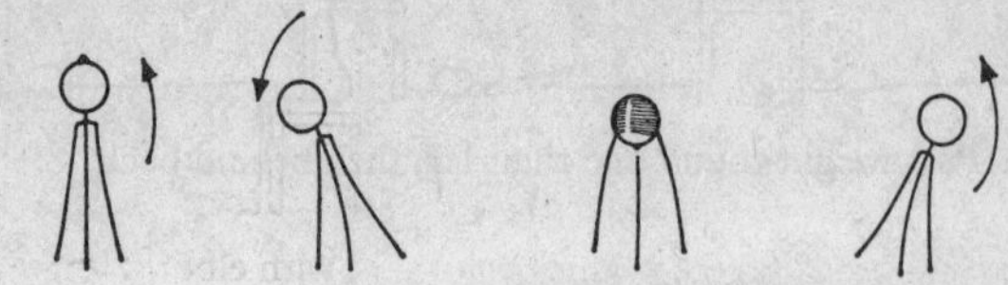

4. Circle head slowly to the right, then to the left. Relax shoulders, keep tummy in

Ribcage and Back Exercises

Fig. 56

To mobilize thorax and spine and firm waistline. Breathe
naturally and easily. Follow movements to music, 4 beats per
picture.

*Starting
position*

1. Turn as far as you can to the right and then to the left – look
behind you each time

Sit correctly. See
sitting posture.
Head up, sit tall,
with hands behind
head, elbows back,
feet on floor, hips
well back in chair.
Relax shoulders.
Long neck

2. Bend sideways to the right, then the left. Keep your head back
and shoulders down

3. Lift alternate knee to opposite elbow

4. Round your back with elbows forward, press back into chair.
Then arch your back, with elbows back

Chest and Breast Exercises

Fig. 57

Exercise to strengthen muscles round the ribcage.
Breathe naturally and easily. Hold position and count for 4 – no
movement takes place – then relax for 4.

Starting position

1. Place hands on top of thighs, press down as hard as you can, and hold for four counts

Sit well back in chair. Keep head up, shoulders back. Long neck. Sit tall, with knees together, thighs on seat. Feet together

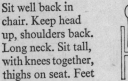

2. Place fists inside thighs – press outwards. Place fists outside thighs – press inwards

3. Push hands together, grip fingers and pull hands apart. Do exercise below and above head

4. Place one hand on top of the other – press together. Change hands

Shoulder-girdle Exercises

Fig. 58

To relieve tension and stiffness in shoulders. Do movements
slowly and continuously. Follow to music, 4 beats per picture.

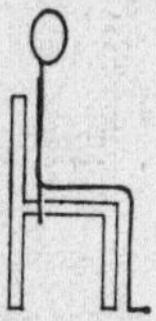

*Starting
position*

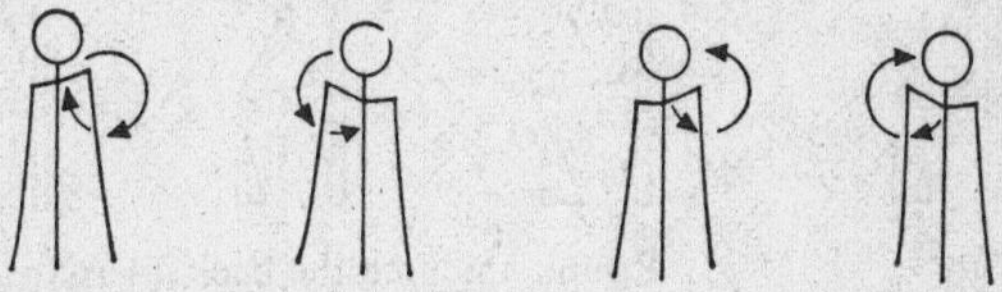

1. Circle alternate shoulders forwards. Circle alternate shoulders
   backwards

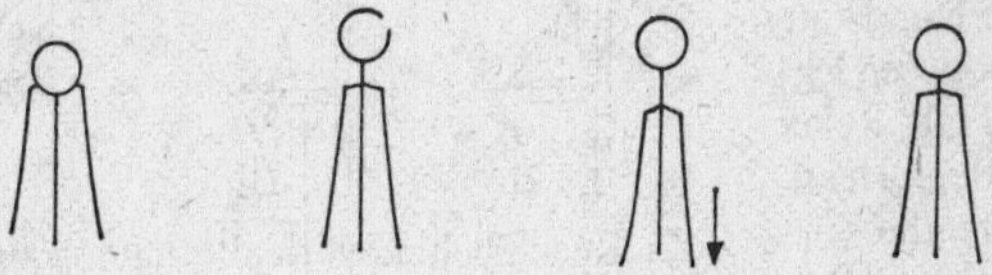

Sit up tall. Head up
and still. Chin in.
Relax shoulders.
Arms relaxed.
Breathe easily.
Long neck

2. Lift both shoulders up to ears. Relax halfway. Press both
   shoulders down hard

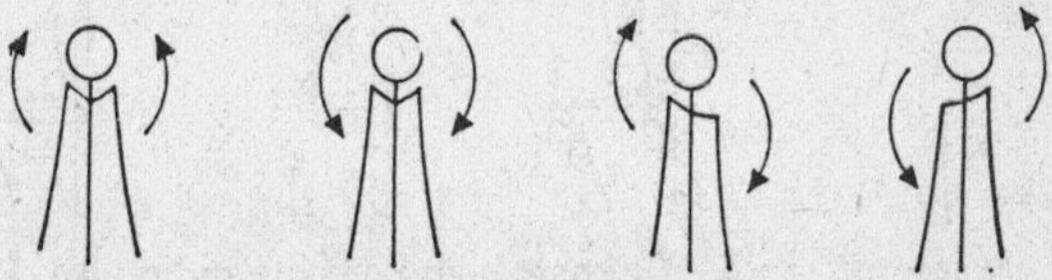

3. Circle both shoulders forwards then backwards. Circle
   shoulders one after the other, in figure eight

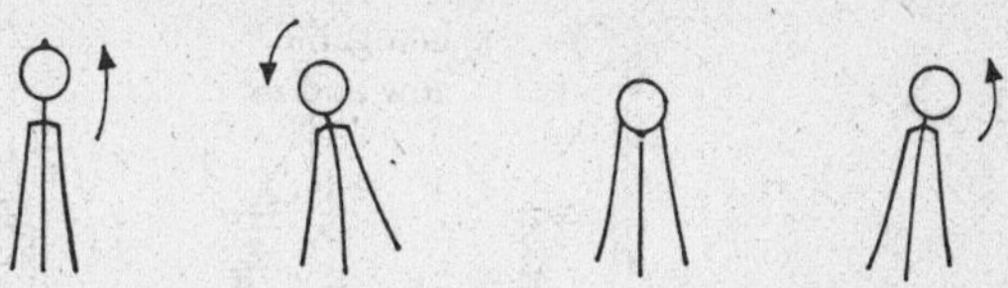

4. Relaxed, head rolling to right in circles. Relaxed, head rolling
   to left

Spine and Hip Exercises

Fig. 59

To mobilize the spine and hips. Do movements slowly and stretch fully. Fit into music, 4 beats per picture.

Starting position

1. Round and arch the back alternately, chin into chest and up to ceiling

Sit forward in chair. Knees wide apart. Hands on seat between legs. Sit up tall. Relax shoulders. Head up. Breathe naturally. Pull up pelvic-floor muscles inside

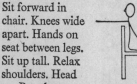

2. Reach behind with alternate straight arm – look at hand as you turn

3. Alternate high-knee lift and return. Roll hips back into chair, when knee is raised

4. Press both knees wide apart and relax

Shoulder and Thigh Exercises

Fig. 60

Exercises to strengthen muscles. Keep breathing normally,
throughout. No movement takes place, hold position and count
to four. The person in chair is working. Partner resists.

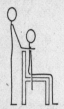 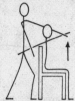

*Starting
position*

Sit well back in
chair. Sit tall.
Relax shoulders.
Head up. Feet firm.
Keep breathing.
Standing partner
keep back straight.
When resisting,
have wide base.
Bend knees, not
back

1. Sitter press arms upwards and hold for four. Sitter press arms
   downwards and hold. Partner resists. Change places

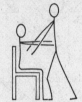 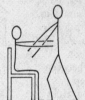

2. Sitter press arms outwards and hold for four. Sitter press
   arms inwards and hold. Partner resists. Change places

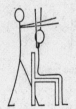 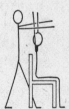

3. Sitter press arms inwards and hold. Sitter press arms
   outwards and hold. Partner resists. Change places

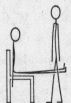 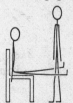

4. Sitter press legs outwards and hold. Sitter press legs inwards
   and hold. Partner resists. Change places

Knee-joint and Thigh-muscle Exercises

Fig. 61

To mobilize the knee joint and strengthen the thigh muscles.
Follow to music, 4 beats per picture.

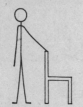
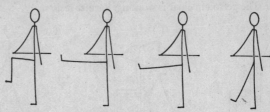

Starting position

1. Bend leg, stretch, hold stretched, lower. Alternate legs

Stand tall. Weight over ankles. Tuck tail in. Tummy in. Shoulders down. Head up. Pull up pelvic-floor muscles between legs. Keep breathing. Hold chair lightly.

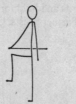
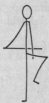
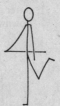
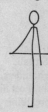

2. Bend leg forwards, sideways, backwards, and return to standing – outside leg only

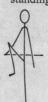
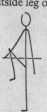
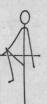
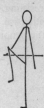

3. Alternate high-knee bending

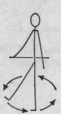
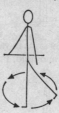
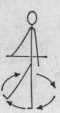
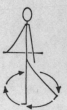

4. Swing full circle with outside leg only. Forwards, sideways, backwards and down. Change sides and repeat

Hip and Pelvic-girdle Exercises

Fig. 62

To mobilize hip joints and strengthen muscles around pelvis. Fit the movements to music, 4 beats per picture.

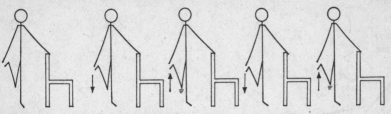

Starting position

1. Keeping one leg straight – lower and lift bent leg. Change Legs

Stand up tall. Bend outside knee. Thighs parallel. Knees touching. Pelvis straight. Tummy in. Head up. Shoulders down. Tuck tail in. Keep breathing

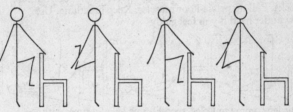

2. Swing bent knee forwards and backwards. Keep back straight – change legs

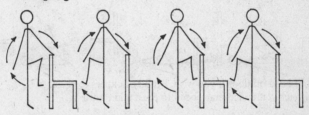

3. Swing bent knee full circle – forwards, sideways, backwards and down. Outside leg only

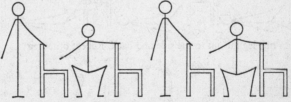

4. Heels together, bend knees as low as you can. Up on toes

Abdominal Muscle Exercises

Fig. 63

For strengthening and firming tummy muscles. Put into sequence, to music, 4 beats per picture. Keep breathing throughout exercises.

Starting position

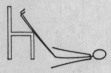

Press back into floor. Harden tummy before lifting legs. Squeeze buttocks. Pull up pelvic-floor muscles. Keep breathing. Use pillow under head if you feel giddy

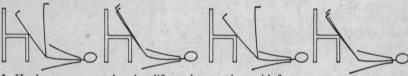

1. Harden tummy muscles, then lift one leg at a time, with feet turned up. Breathe naturally

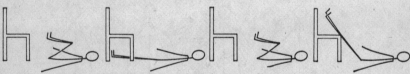

2. Lift head off floor if you wish, bend both knees to chest. Stretch out under chair, bend to chest and return

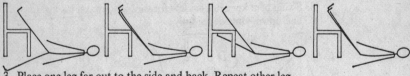

3. Place one leg far out to the side and back. Repeat other leg

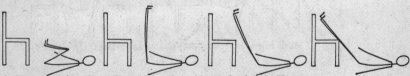

4. Press back into floor. Bend, stretch and lower both legs. Keep breathing

Trunk-muscle Exercises

Fig. 64

To strengthen abdominal and back muscles. Good for the
waistline and spare tyre. Fit movements to music, 4 beats per
picture.

*Starting
position*

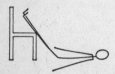

Firm tummy. Harden buttocks. Press neck down. Pull up pelvic-
floor muscles. Keep breathing. Use pillow under head if you wish

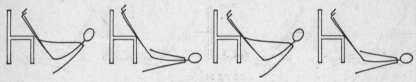

1. Right hand to left knee – repeat other hand

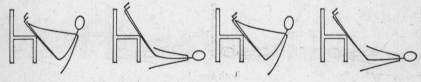

2. Right hand to left foot – repeat other side

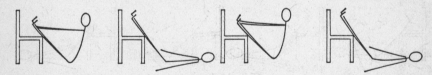

3. Both hands to both feet – uncurl back to floor

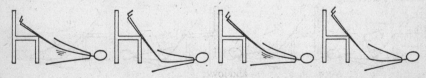

4. Hips lift and lower slowly

Hip-joint Exercises

Fig. 65

To mobilize the hip joint and strengthen and firm surrounding muscles. Fit movements into sequence and to music, 4 beats per picture.

Starting
position

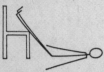

Never fall asleep in this position unless support given under knees. Harden abdominals. Keep breathing. Relax shoulders. Long neck. Firm buttocks and pelvic-floor muscles

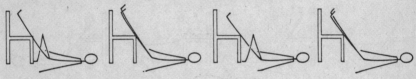

1. Cross one leg over the other, touch floor with foot

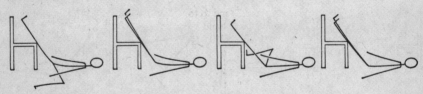

2. Bend one leg out sideways and touch floor

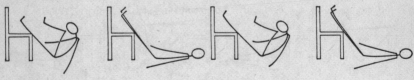

3. Bend alternate knee and touch forehead. Relax between each. Keep breathing

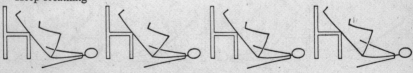

4. Legs cycling at chair height, firm abdominal muscles before starting. Breathe naturally

Upper Spine and Shoulder Exercises

Fig. 66

To mobilize spine and strengthen muscles of the shoulder girdle.
Fit movements into sequence, 4 beats per picture.

*Starting
position*

Head between arms. Nose on floor. Buttocks raised. Relax
shoulders. Keep breathing. Reach forward with hands. Tummy in

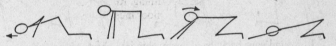

1. Gently press shoulders towards floor

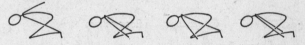

2. Run nose along floor between hands, lift head and body, and
    back to start

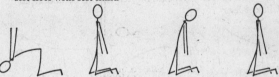

3. Keep low, side bend to touch right heel with right hand, then
    left heel with left hand

4. Knees slightly apart, round and arch back alternately

Spine and Hip Exercises

Fig. 67

To mobilize the joints of the spine and hips. Follow sequence,
4 beats per picture.

*Starting
position*

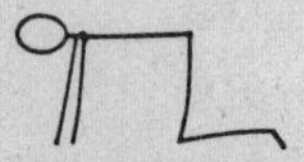

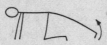

Hands directly under shoulders. Tummy in. Long neck. Cushion
for knees if required. If wrists hurt lean on elbows or fists.
Breathe naturally

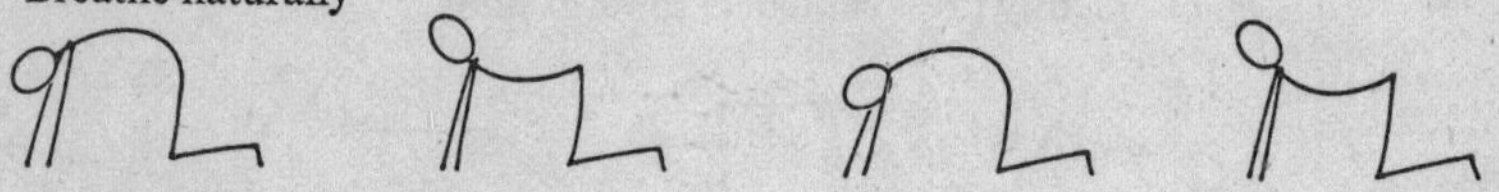

1. Round your back, head down, chin into chest. Arch your
   back, head up. Hump and arch

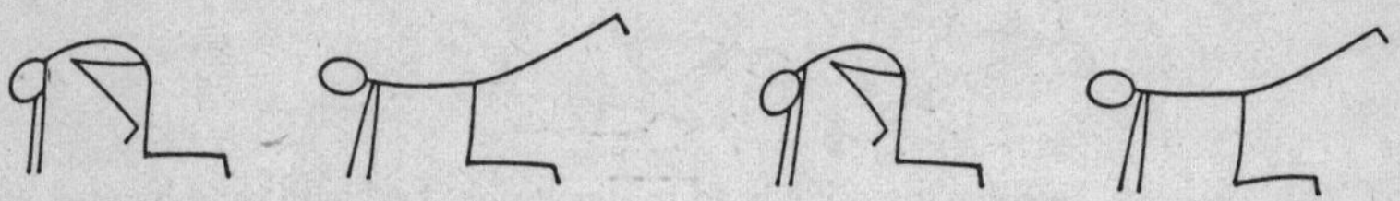

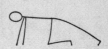

2. Bend knee, touch forehead. Stretch leg out behind, head up.
   Change legs

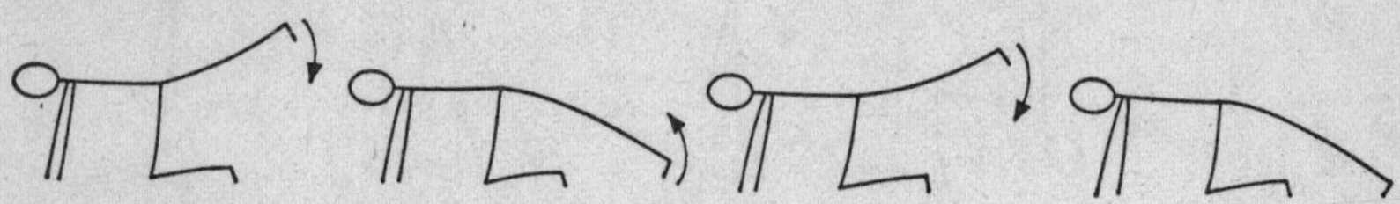

3. Make a large circle with one straight leg. Change legs and
   direction

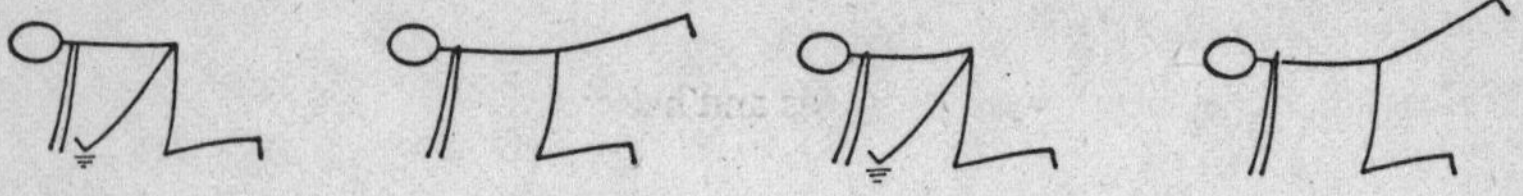

4. Swing leg sideways and back

Hip Exercises

Fig. 68

To strengthen buttocks and thigh muscles and mobilize hip joint.
Put movements to music, 4 beats per picture.

*Starting
position*

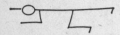

Side-lying. Rest head on arm. Under leg bent. Relax head and
shoulders. Breathe easily. Tummy firm. Buttocks firm. Keep feet
turned up, ankles towards ceiling

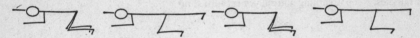

1. Bend and stretch top leg

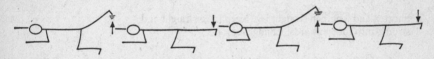

2. Lift straight top leg, up and down, away from floor

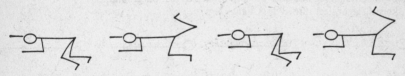

3. Keeping top leg bent, swing forwards and backwards

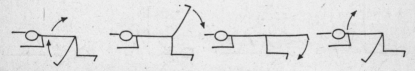

4. Circle straight top leg. Change sides and start again

More Hip Exercises

Fig. 69

To mobilize hip joints and strengthen thigh muscles. Fit
movements to music, 4 beats per picture.

*Starting
position*

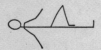

Half crook-lying. Press back into floor. Firm tummy. Relax
shoulders. Long neck. Firm buttocks. Pull up pelvic-floor
muscles. Keep breathing naturally. Feet turned up

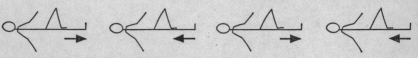

1. Shorten and lengthen straight leg. Keep knee straight and
   strong, turn foot upwards. Change legs

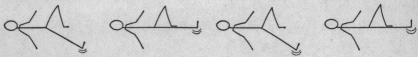

2. Swing straight leg out sideways and back. Leg just off ground,
   knee straight, feet turned up. Change legs

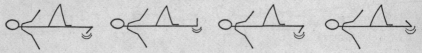

3. Turn leg outwards and inwards – leg just off ground, knee
   straight, feet turned up. Change legs

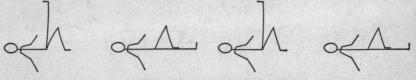

4. Lift leg straight up and down slowly. Feet turned up. Change
   legs

Abdominal Muscle Exercises

Fig. 70

To strengthen abdominal muscles and mobilize spine, hip and knee joints. Put into sequence, to music, 4 beats per picture.

Starting
position

Crook-lying. Harden tummy. Press back into floor. Firm buttocks. Relax shoulders. Long neck. Pull up pelvic-floor muscles. Keep breathing easily. Lie on mat if required. Pillow under head if desired

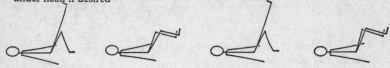

1. Straighten alternate legs, change in mid-air. Press back into floor, keep breathing. Tap mat with alternate feet. Keep knees together

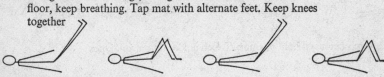

2. Straighten both legs to angle of 45° to floor and return. Firm tummy. Keep breathing

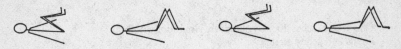

3. Knees bend to chest and lower feet to floor. Keep legs bent all the time. Breathe naturally

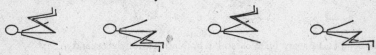

4. Knees bend to chest, lower to one side, then the other. Keep both shoulders on floor

Hip Mobility Exercises

Fig. 71

To loosen and relax muscles, joints and ligaments around the hip area. Put movement to music, 4 beats per picture.

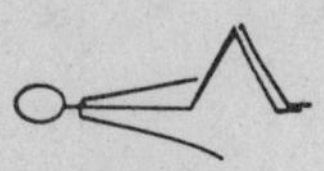

Crook-lying. Knees together. Feet apart. Press back into floor. Relax shoulders. Firm buttocks. Long neck. Keep breathing

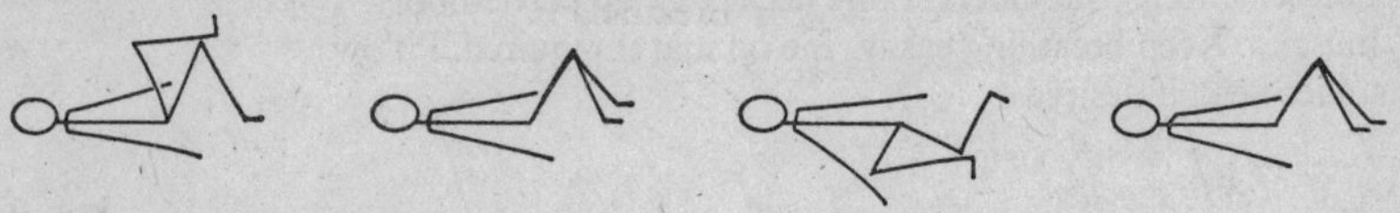

1. Drop both knees to left side so that the right knee touches left heel. Repeat other side

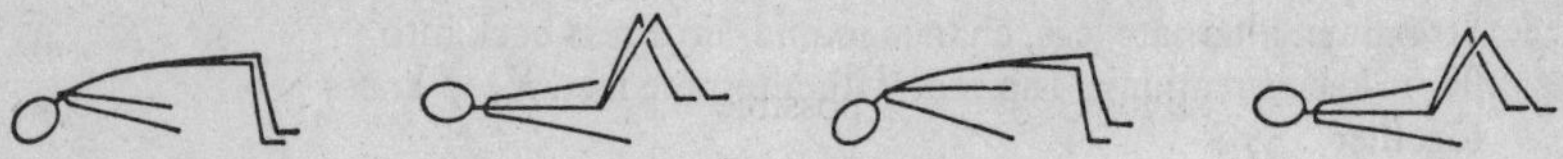

2. Arch back and hold position. Touch ankles if you can. Open knees slightly

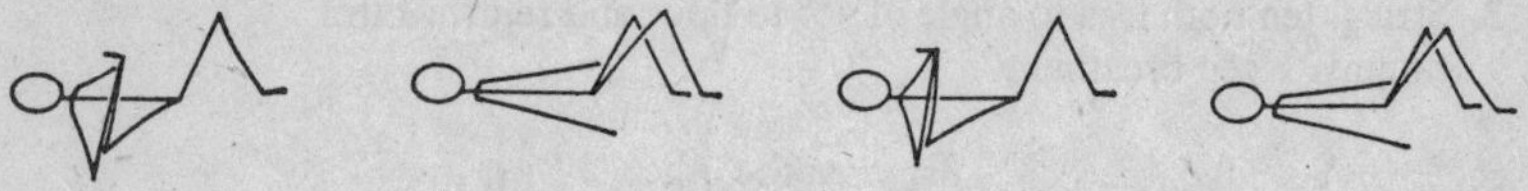

3. One knee touches floor by shoulder. Hold foot with both hands and gently stretch

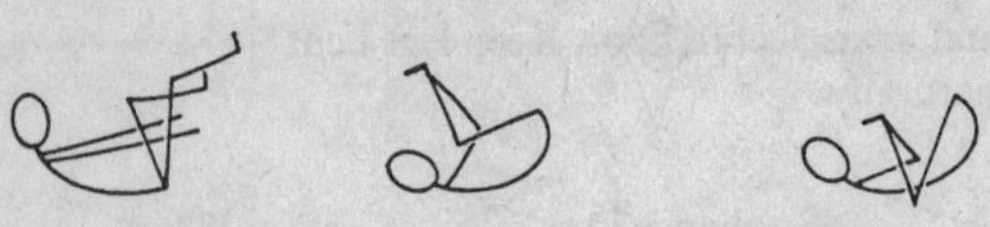

4. Bend knees apart, up to chest. Put both arms through legs and grip ankles. Gently pull both knees to floor either side of body

Hip and Buttock Exercises

Fig. 72

To strengthen buttocks and loosen stiff hips and knee joints. Fit to music. Follow sequence, 4 beats per picture.

Starting position

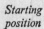

Prone-lying. Rest forehead on hands. Breathe easily. Relax shoulders. Firm tummy and buttocks

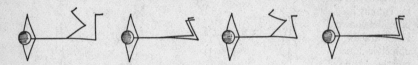

1 Lift alternate bent legs as high as possible

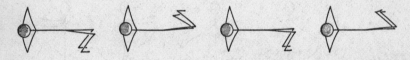

2. Drop both bent legs one side, then the other. Touch the floor each time with feet

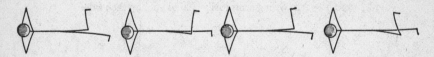

3. Straighten alternate legs to floor, change in mid-air. (Double time)

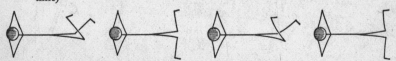

4. Cross legs behind and part. (Double time)

Free-standing Exercises

Fig. 73

General exercises to relieve tension and feel stretched and upright before relaxation. Put movements to music.

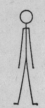

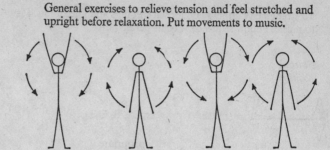

Starting position

Standing feet slightly apart for balance. Tuck tail in. Tummy in. Shoulders down. Head straight. Pull up pelvic-floor muscles. Lean weight over ankles. Grow tall. Keep breathing

1. Both arms slowly circling above head and down to sides. Brush ears with upper arm. Go up on toes and down

 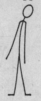

2. Side bending slowly – alternate sides

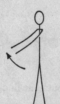 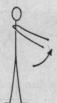 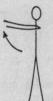 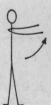

3. Swing arms easily behind you, on each side

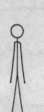 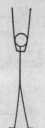 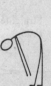

4. Reach for your toes and stretch up tall. Now get ready for the relaxation

Appendix 1
The Fitness Circuit Chart (see Figs. 51–4)

Choose 4 exercises – 1 each from Parts A, B, C, D.
Tick the exercise you have chosen.
Fill in the number of times for the appropriate duration.
Record on chart every day.

	Number of Times			*Notes*
	½ *Minute every day*	*1 Minute every day*	*1½ Minutes every day*	
	Week I	Week II	Week III onwards	
Part A Ex. 1 2 3 4				
Part B Ex. 1 2 3 4				
Part C Ex. 1 2 3 4				
Part D Ex. 1 2 3 4				

Appendix 2
Approximate Number of Calories *Per Day* Needed at Different Life Stages

Sex	Years of Age	Strength of Activity	Weight of body st lb		Calories
Boys	9–12	Moderate to strong	5	0	2,500
Boys	12–15	Moderate to strong	7	2	2,800
Boys	15–18	Moderate to strong	9	8	3,000
Girls	9–12	Moderate to strong	5	3	2,300
Girls	12–15	Moderate to strong	7	9	2,300
Girls	15–18	Moderate to strong	8	12	2,300
Men	18–35	Light	10	3	2,700
Men	18–35	Moderate	10	3	3,000
Men	18–35	Strenuous	10	3	3,600
Men	18–35	Very strenuous	10	3	4,200
Men	35–65	Light	10	3	2,600
Men	35–65	Moderate	10	3	2,900
Men	35–65	Strenuous	10	3	3,600
Men	65–75	Light	9	13	2,350
Men	75 and over	Light	9	13	2,100
Women	18–55	Moderate	8	9	2,200
Women	18–55	Strenuous	8	9	2,500
Women	55–75	Light to moderate	8	5	2,050
Women	75 and over	Light	8	5	1,900

The heavier you are the more energy you use for the same activity.

Appendix 3
Approximate Number of Calories *Per Minute* Needed for Various Activities

1. *Sleeping* (1 calorie per minute)
2. *Sitting and standing* (1–2 calories per minute)
3. *Light activities* (approximately 2–5 calories per minute)

Bowling	Knitting	Walking slowly
Classwork	Playing cards	Washing a car
Cooking	Preparing meals	Washing up
Dressing	Reading	Washing yourself, etc.
Driving a car	Sewing	
Dusting	Typing	

4. *Moderate activities* (approximately 5–10 calories per minute)

Ballroom dancing	Golf	Some gardening
Baseball	Housework	Swimming
Carpentry	Jogging	Tennis
Cricket	Polishing	Walking fast
Cycling	Sailing	Walking up and down
Decorating	Scrubbing	stairs
D.I.Y.	Shopping (heavy load)	Window cleaning, etc.

5. *Strenuous and very strenuous activities* (approximately 10–20 calories per minute)

Athletics	Digging	Pot holing
Ballet	Football	Running
Baseball Pitcher	Gym exercises	Running up and down
Basket Ball	Heavy gardening	stairs
Canoeing	Hill climbing	Sawing by hand
Climbing	Mining	Skiing
Cross-country running	Netball	Squash
		Swimming (free style, etc.)

Appendix 4
Personal Statistics Chart

	First Week	Fifth Week	Tenth Week
Bust			
Waist			
Hips			
Thighs			
Height			
Weight			
Weight Aim			
Frame S.M.L.			
Ideal Weight Range			
Weight Loss			
Measurement Loss			

Appendix 5
Ideal-weight Charts

(Reprinted from Metropolitan Life Insurance Company Stat. Bull. 40: 1–12 (Nov. Dec.) 1959)

WOMEN (aged 25 years or more)

Height in Shoes ft in	Small Frame st lb st lb	Medium Frame st lb st lb	Large Frame st lb st lb
4 10	6 8– 7 0	6 12– 7 9	7 6– 8 7
4 11	6 10– 7 3	7 0– 7 12	7 8– 8 10
5 0	6 12– 7 6	7 3– 8 1	7 11– 8 13
5 1	7 1– 7 9	7 6– 8 4	8 0– 9 2
5 2	7 4– 7 12	7 9– 8 7	8 3– 9 5
5 3	7 7– 8 1	7 12– 8 10	8 6– 9 8
5 4	7 10– 8 4	8 1– 9 0	8 9– 9 12
5 5	7 13– 8 7	8 4– 9 4	8 13–10 2
5 6	8 2– 8 11	8 8– 9 9	9 3–10 6
5 7	8 6– 9 1	8 12– 9 13	9 7–10 10
5 8	8 10– 9 5	9 2–10 3	9 11–11 0
5 9	9 0– 9 9	9 6–10 7	10 1–11 4
5 10	9 4–10 0	9 10–10 11	10 5–11 9
5 11	9 8–10 4	10 0–11 1	10 9–12 0
6 0	9 12–10 8	10 4–11 5	10 13–12 5

MEN (aged 25 years or more)

Height in Shoes ft in	Small Frame st lb st lb	Medium Frame st lb st lb	Large Frame st lb st lb
5 2	8 0– 8 8	8 6– 9 3	9 0–10 1
5 3	8 3– 8 11	8 9– 9 7	9 3–10 4
5 4	8 6– 9 0	8 12– 9 10	9 6–10 8
5 5	8 9– 9 3	9 1– 9 13	9 9–10 12
5 6	8 12– 9 7	9 4–10 3	9 12–11 2
5 7	9 2– 9 11	9 8–10 7	10 2–11 7
5 8	9 6–10 1	9 12–10 12	10 7–11 12
5 9	9 10–10 5	10 2–11 2	10 11–12 2
5 10	10 0–10 10	10 6–11 6	11 1–12 6
5 11	10 4–11 0	10 10–11 11	11 5–12 11
6 0	10 8–11 4	11 0–12 2	11 10–13 2
6 1	10 12–11 8	11 4–12 7	12 0–13 7
6 2	11 2–11 13	11 8–12 12	12 5–13 12
6 3	11 6–12 3	11 13–13 3	12 10–14 3
6 4	11 10–12 7	12 4–13 8	13 0–14 8

Appendix 6
Conversion Table for Weight

Stones and pounds to kilograms

(Conversions are correct to the nearest 0·1 kg (100 grams); i.e. approximately 3 oz.)

st	lb	kg	st	lb	kg	st	lb	kg	st	lb	kg	st	lb	kg	st	lb	kg
2	0	12·7	5	0	31·8	8	0	50·8	11	0	69·9	14	0	88·9	17	0	107·9
2	1	13·2	5	1	32·2	8	1	51·3	11	1	70·3	14	1	89·4	17	1	108·4
2	2	13·6	5	2	32·7	8	2	51·7	11	2	70·8	14	2	89·8	17	2	108·9
2	3	14·1	5	3	33·1	8	3	52·2	11	3	71·2	14	3	90·3	17	3	109·3
2	4	14·5	5	4	33·6	8	4	52·6	11	4	71·7	14	4	90·7	17	4	109·8
2	5	15·0	5	5	34·0	8	5	53·1	11	5	72·2	14	5	91·2	17	5	110·2
2	6	15·4	5	6	34·5	8	6	53·5	11	6	72·6	14	6	91·6	17	6	110·7
2	7	15·9	5	7	34·9	8	7	54·0	11	7	73·0	14	7	92·1	17	7	111·1
2	8	16·3	5	8	35·4	8	8	54·4	11	8	73·5	14	8	92·5	17	8	111·7
2	9	16·8	5	9	35·8	8	9	54·9	11	9	73·9	14	9	93·0	17	9	112·0
2	10	17·2	5	10	36·3	8	10	55·3	11	10	74·4	14	10	93·4	17	10	112·5
2	11	17·7	5	11	36·7	8	11	55·8	11	11	74·8	14	11	93·9	17	11	112·9
2	12	18·1	5	12	37·2	8	12	56·2	11	12	75·3	14	12	94·3	17	12	113·4
2	13	18·6	5	13	37·6	8	13	56·7	11	13	75·8	14	13	94·8	17	13	113·9
3	0	19·1	6	0	38·1	9	0	57·2	12	0	76·2	15	0	95·2	18	0	114·3
3	1	19·5	6	1	38·6	9	1	57·6	12	1	76·7	15	1	95·7	18	1	114·8

3 2	20·0	6 2	39·0	9 2	58·1	12 2	77·1	15 2	96·2	18 2	115·2
3 3	20·4	6 3	39·5	9 3	58·5	12 3	77·6	15 3	96·6	18 3	115·7
3 4	20·9	6 4	39·9	9 4	59·0	12 4	78·0	15 4	97·0	18 4	116·1
3 5	21·3	6 5	40·4	9 5	59·4	12 5	78·5	15 5	97·5	18 5	116·6
3 6	21·8	6 6	40·8	9 6	59·9	12 6	78·9	15 6	98·0	18 6	117·0
3 7	22·2	6 7	41·3	9 7	60·3	12 7	79·4	15 7	98·4	18 7	117·5
3 8	22·7	6 8	41·7	9 8	60·8	12 8	79·8	15 8	98·9	18 8	117·9
3 9	23·1	6 9	42·2	9 9	61·2	12 9	80·1	15 9	99·3	18 9	118·4
3 10	23·6	6 10	42·6	9 10	61·7	12 10	80·7	15 10	99·8	18 10	118·8
3 11	24·0	6 11	43·1	9 11	62·1	12 11	81·2	15 11	100·2	18 11	119·3
3 12	24·5	6 12	43·5	9 12	62·6	12 12	81·6	15 12	100·7	18 12	119·7
3 13	24·9	6 13	44·0	9 13	63·0	12 13	82·1	15 13	101·2	18 13	120·2
4 0	25·4	7 0	44·5	10 0	63·5	13 0	82·6	16 0	101·6	19 0	120·7
4 1	25·9	7 1	44·9	10 1	64·0	13 1	83·0	16 1	102·1	19 1	121·1
4 2	26·3	7 2	45·4	10 2	64·4	13 2	83·5	16 2	102·5	19 2	121·6
4 3	26·8	7 3	45·8	10 3	64·9	13 3	83·9	16 3	103·0	19 3	122·0
4 4	27·2	7 4	46·3	10 4	65·3	13 4	84·4	16 4	103·4	19 4	122·5
4 5	27·7	7 5	46·7	10 5	65·8	13 5	84·8	16 5	103·9	19 5	122·9
4 6	28·1	7 6	47·2	10 6	66·2	13 6	85·3	16 6	104·3	19 6	123·4
4 7	28·6	7 7	47·6	10 7	66·7	13 7	85·7	16 7	194·8	19 7	123·8
4 8	29·0	7 8	48·1	10 8	67·1	13 8	86·2	16 8	105·2	19 8	124·3
4 9	29·5	7 9	48·5	10 9	67·6	13 9	86·6	16 9	105·7	19 9	124·7
4 10	29·9	7 10	49·0	10 10	68·0	13 10	87·1	16 10	106·1	19 10	125·2
4 11	30·4	7 11	49·4	10 11	68·5	13 11	87·5	16 11	106·6	19 11	125·6
4 12	30·8	7 12	49·9	10 12	68·9	13 12	88·0	16 12	107·0	19 12	126·1
4 13	31·3	7 13	50·3	10 13	69·4	13 13	88·5	16 13	107·5	19 13	126·6
										20 00	127·0

Appendix 7
Your Personal Diet Sheet

Fill in all your food and drink intake for one week.

Date	Morning	Afternoon	Evening	Parties Illness Excuses!

More About Penguins and Pelicans

Penguinews, which appears every month, contains details of all the new books issued by Penguins as they are published. It is supplemented by our stocklist, which includes almost 5,000 titles.

A specimen copy of *Penguinews* will be sent to you free on request. Please write to Dept EP, Penguin Books Ltd, Harmondsworth, Middlesex, for your copy.

In the U.S.A.: For a complete list of books available from Penguins in the United States write to Dept CS, Penguin Books, 625 Madison Avenue, New York, New York 10022.

In Canada: For a complete list of books available from Penguins in Canada write to Penguin Books Canada Ltd, 2801 John Street, Markham, Ontario L3R 1B4.

In Australia: For a complete list of books published by Penguins in Australia write to the Marketing Department, Penguin Books Australia Ltd, P.O. Box 257, Ringwood, Victoria 3134.

How to Lose Weight Without Really Dieting

Michael Spira

1. Lose weight without crash dieting, counting calories or feeling hungry and irritable.
2. Re-educate yourself so that you are both slim *and* healthy.
3. Eat your favourite cream bun and still keep the svelte outline – whatever your age.
4. Learn about the constituents of food and how they affect weight and health.

How to Lose Weight Without Really Dieting
debunks current slimming fads and fallacies, offering instead a sensible scientifically based programme of eating that will help even the weakest willed to take off weight. Michael Spira realizes that if you love rice pudding you are not likely to really give it up and, taking this into account, he shows you how to establish successful eating patterns which, with only a little self-control, will last you for the rest of your life.

In short, Dr Spira tells you how to have your cake and eat it.

The Exercise Book

Leslie Michener and Gerald Donaldson

If you want every inch of your body to look and feel its best here's the book that shows you how – clearly, simply, beautifully.

Whatever your present shape or level of fitness, you can use this portable, scientifically-devised physical fitness programme.

You don't need any special equipment or time-consuming trips to a gym.

The Exercise Book involves nearly every muscle in the body and can be used by anyone, anywhere, at any time.

Your instructor is Leslie Michener, a physical education professional. Over 400 colour and black-and-white photographs show her demonstrating the 48 Movement Patterns that make up the complete programme. Every step of the way is fully illustrated and described.

This Slimming Business

John Yudkin

John Yudkin, Professor of Nutrition and Dietetics in the University of London, here gives authoritative advice about slimming and how to draw the lines between fact, fashion, and fad.

Although a good deal of nonsense is printed in some women's magazines about slimming, Professor Yudkin shows in this readable and often entertaining handbook that the effort involved in carrying extra weight can be harmful and may lead to a number of ailments, some fatal. For other than merely fashionable reasons, therefore, it is wise to watch your weight – without being too impressed by the so-called average weight tables – and, if necessary, to take sensible steps to reduce it.

This Slimming Business is not heavy reading. Light verses by Ogden Nash help the author's easy style to keep the weight well down.

The Slimmer's Cookbook

John Yudkin and Gweneth M. Chappell

The best diet for slimming is also the best diet for health. In this book Professor Yudkin and Gweneth M. Chappell, a senior lecturer in Household Science, present the would-be slimmer with a selection of dishes which ensure that he or she need never feel hungry. The preparation of these is based on the principle of cutting down as much as possible on the intake of carbohydrates, replacing them with meat, fish, eggs, and all the other protein-giving foods. Contrary to popular belief, the cost of these foods is not prohibitive: a wide range of inexpensive dishes is described. In addition to more simple meals which can be prepared in a matter of minutes, there are also many elaborate concoctions for social occasions, suitable for slimmers and non-slimmers alike. A special section on 'portable' low-carbohydrate meals is included for those who daily take packed lunches to their place of work. This new edition includes a valuable table of carbohydrate units.